BREATHING
FREE

BREATHING FREE

The Revolutionary 5-Day Program to Heal
Asthma, Emphysema, Bronchitis,
and Other Respiratory Ailments

TERESA HALE

FOREWORD BY LEO GALLAND, M.D.

Harmony Books
New York

This book is intended as a guide to people who want to improve and maintain their health. If you are concerned in any way about your health, you should seek medical advice.

Published by Harmony Books, 201 East 50th Street, New York, New York 10022. Member of the Crown Publishing Group.

Originally published in Great Britain by Hodder and Stoughton in 1999.

Random House, Inc. New York, Toronto, London, Sydney, Auckland www.randomhouse.com

HARMONY BOOKS is a registered trademark and Harmony Books colophon is a trademark of Random House, Inc.

Printed in the United States of America

Library of Congress Cataloging-in-Publication Data
Hale, Teresa.
Breathing free : the revolutionary 5 day program to heal asthma, emphysema, bronchitis, and other respiratory ailments / Teresa Hale.
p.   cm.
Includes bibliographical references and index.
1. Respiratory organs—Diseases—Treatment.   2. Breathing exercises.   I. Title.

RC731.H34   1999   99-30267
616.2'0046—dc21   CIP

ISBN 0-609-60424-4

10   9   8   7   6   5   4   3   2   1

First American Edition

*To my mother Vee Hale,
my late father William Hale,
and my grandfather Alfred Steel,
who suffered from asthma
and could never breathe freely.*

Contents

Contents

Contents

CONTENTS

CONTENTS

Foreword

LEO GALLAND, M.D.,
Director, Foundation for Integrated Medicine

Techniques of breathing are of great importance in many traditional healing systems, especially those of India and China, where healers believed that how you breathe influences your health. Modern Western doctors, in contrast, emphasize the effect of health on breath. If you breathe abnormally, it is because you have a disease. In the December 1998 issue of *The New Republic,* the editor of the prestigious *New England Journal of Medicine* launched a caustic attack on alternative medicine by stating that your health determines how you breathe, but how you breathe has no effect on your state of health. Despite his protestations, there is considerable sicentific evidence that how you breathe impacts on your health. Not only does health affect breath, breath affects health as well.

The main reason for breathing, of course, is to replenish your body's supply of oxygen. If your lungs are healthy, obtaining oxygen from the air is rarely a problem. The complex effects of breathing on health have less to do with oxygen than with *carbon dioxide.* We're taught that carbon dioxide is a waste product, the final result of the burning of fuel in the body, a gas that we expel each time we breathe out. However, carbon dioxide is much more. It is a chemical that regulates the acid-alkaline balance of your blood and of your cells. An excess of carbon dioxide in your blood causes an excess of acidity. A deficiency of carbon dioxide produces a state of excessive alkalinity. Because the main route for eliminating carbon dioxide from your body is the lungs, how you breathe affects the carbon dioxide level in your blood. Severe lung disease produces an excess of carbon dioxide by interfering with its elimination. Far more common are deficiencies of carbon dioxide that result from overbreathing, a condition called "hyperventilation." Hyperventilation may result from anxiety or more commonly from acquired habits of breathing that may be shaped by chronic stress.

The effects of hyperventilation on the body are well-known. The increase in alkalinity of the blood causes both calcium and magnesium in the circulation to become attached to the blood's major protein, albumen. This protein-binding lowers the level of free calcium and magnesium, creating a virtual deficiency of these important minerals. The major consequence is muscle spasm that affects both the voluntary muscles that permit you to move and the involuntary muscles that line the arteries, the intestines and the bronchial tubes. Spasm of the voluntary muscles may produce pain and stiffness. Spasm of the involuntary muscles may cause narrowing of the blood vessels and the bronchial tubes and cramping of the intestines. Narrowing of the blood vessels interferes with blood flow to many parts of your body. It may produce cold hands and feet, chest pains and palpitations, dizziness and difficulty with concentration. Spasm of the bronchial tubes may cause shortness of breath.

These effects of carbon dioxide deficiency are aggravated by another effect of carbon dioxide: its influence on the way in which oxygen is carried by the blood. Oxygen is transported from the lungs to the cells of your body in the red blood cells, where it is bound to hemoglobin, a protein that gives blood its red color. When the blood is excessively acid, hemoglobin gives up its oxygen more readily, making it more accessible to your body's cells. When the blood is excessively alkaline (when there is a deficiency of carbon dioxide, that is), hemoglobin is *less able* to release oxygen to your cells. The result is a relative deficiency of oxygen.

Carbon dioxide deficiency, therefore, can wreak havoc with the normal functioning of your body by preventing calcium, magnesium and oxygen from reaching the cells. These facts are undisputed. There is no controversy about them. Controversy surrounds the questions, How common is this condition? How often does it produce ill health? What role does it play in diseases like asthma, migraine headaches and panic disorder?

In the United States most doctors have believed that hyperventilation only occurs as an acute, dramatic illness that is the result of anxiety and that produces dizziness, breathlessness, numbness and tingling of the mouth and the hands, creating more anxiety. In Europe, on the other hand, researchers have described a state known as *chronic hyperventilation,* in which a person's habitual pattern of breathing causes a chronic deficiency of carbon dioxide and chronic, fluctuating symptoms that may involve any or all of the body's muscles. Chronic hyperventilation may cause dizziness, lightheadedness, fatigue, muscle tension, muscle cramps, intestinal or bladder spasms, palpitations, chest pains, and headache. Strangely enough, chronic hyperventilation also creates a shortness of breath, which leads to more hyperventilation, producing a vicious cycle. The shortness of breath resulting from hyperventilation may have three causes: (1) a decrease in blood flow to certain parts of the brain resulting from spasm of blood vessels in the brain; (2) spasm of the bronchial muscles which narrows the air passages to the lungs; and (3) decreased release of oxygen to the cells of the body, even though the oxygen level in the blood appears normal. There have been different approaches to solving the problems caused by chronic hyperventilation: training in a variety of breathing techniques, breathing into a paper bag so that the carbon dioxide you expel with each breath is breathed back in, vigorous exercise to increase the production of acid in the body, magnesium and/or calcium pills, relaxation and stress management training, and even sedative drugs.

Teresa Hale brings to our attention a revolutionary, modern technique of breath control, developed by the Russian physician Konstantin Buteyko. Buteyko was researching the breathing problems of people with asthma, a disorder that has increased dramatically in the past fifty years. He discovered that people with asthma frequently hyperventilate. This observation was not a surprise. Every emergency room doctor knows that many patients with asthma become more and more short of breath the harder they breathe. For these patients breathing more slowly and less deeply is essential for asthma control. Butekyo, however, reached a profound conclusion from this obervation. He surmised that hyperventilation was the *primary* cause of asthma, that the lungs of asthmatics responded to chronic overbreathing with spasm and swelling of the bronchial tubes. His theory extended the impact of hyperventilation beyond its known ability to cause muscle spasm. He believed that asthma was the body's attempt to compensate for the loss of carbon dioxide by making breathing more difficult. He developed a therapy based upon progressive training in breathing less while doing more. This book describes his theory in detail and provides the reader with comprehensive instructions for learning and utilizing Buteyko's technique. Even if the theory is wrong, the technique itself is valuable and has been shown in controlled clinical research conducted in Europe and Australia to improve the symptoms of people with asthma, to increase their capacity for exercise and to decrease their need for medication.

One important component of the Breath Connection program is that the dramatic improvement made to your respiration will enable you to avoid drugs that artificially dilate the bronchial tubes (bronchodilators). In my recent book, *Power Healing* (Random House, 1988), I warned of the dangers of bronchodilator drugs, which are usually taken as inhaled sprays. When these drugs were first used in the 1940s, the death rate from asthma immediately increased. Research during the 1980s revealed that continuous use of bronchodilators was associated with deteriorating lung function and an increased death rate. Respiratory therapists, who are routinely exposed to bronchodilator mists in the course of their work, develop asthma at a rate four times greater than would be expected *after entering their profession*. The adverse outcome of continuous bronchodilation indicates that bronchial spasm is indeed part of a protective response that bronchodilation prevents. Conventional treatment strategies for asthma are a disaster and the Buteyko program is part of the solution.

For those people who suffer from the other effects of chronic hyperventilation, whether asthma is part of the problem or not, the Buteyko program provides a structured and effective method of breath control, which may be of great benefit, especially when incorporated into a comprehensive approach to health restoration that include sound nutrition, regular physical exercise, effective stress management and the cultivation of a healthy physical and social environment. *Breathing Free* presents a welcome addition to the arsenal of holistic and complementary therapies available in the United States today.

Acknowledgments

Professor Konstantin Buteyko, whose discovery linking our breathing patterns to so many diseases became the inspiration behind this book.

My literary agent, Al Lowman, an asthma/emphysema sufferer whose life was transformed by the Breath Connection Program. It was his vision, dogged persistence, and encouragement that resulted in this book being written.

Chip Gibson, the president and publisher of Crown, whose insight and courage was a vital ingredient in the publication of this book.

The patience and commitment of Doug Pepper, my editor at Crown, was greatly appreciated.

My eternal gratitude to Susan Hill, whose inspired editorial skills enabled the content of this book to be expressed so clearly.

Ralph Morris, Danielle Braender, Bianca Foot, and all the administration team at the Hale Clinic, whose hard work provided me with the time in which I could write *Breathing Free*.

Rodney Paul, who portrayed the Breath Connection exercises so well in diagrammatic form.

Finally, my deepest thanks to Sue Carter, who was able to type the manuscript from my illegible writing, which even I can't read.

Introduction

Asthma kills thousands of people every year. Millions of others are severely debilitated by related respiratory illnesses every day of their lives. And asthma is on the increase—it is now the only disease in the Western world that is increasing in epidemic proportions. Perhaps most frightening, modern medicine practices have done nothing to reduce the number of asthma-related deaths, and we are no closer to a cure than we were forty years ago. Over that time, the number of cases, and the number of deaths, has continued to rise. Doctors have little idea of how to prevent this disease, and its cause has remained one of medicine's modern mysteries.

But there is hope. This book introduces a program that will dramatically reduce the symptoms of all asthmatics and anyone suffering from bronchial disorders within as little as five days. By following the program, you can improve your health without the need for drugs or any of the traditional methods used to treat respiratory conditions. Most important, you will make fundamental changes to the way your body works, and, over time, all kinds of niggling health problems will be addressed.

This program involves learning to breathe. Across time, we have been led to believe that deep breathing is good for us because it increases our oxygen intake. In fact, the reverse is true. The more we breathe, the less oxygen actually reaches the cells of our bodies.

Breath Is Life

Gentle, regular breathing is a reassuring sign of peace and healthy rest. Most of us consider the calm rise and fall of the chest, the soft, steady rhythms of breathing itself, to be evidence of good health. Indeed, the physical act of breathing indicates that we are alive. It's not surprising, therefore, that people find it difficult to understand the concept that breathing shouldn't be an obvious function. When we breathe correctly, our chests do not expand and sink. Healthy breathing is quiet and shallow, and our chests barely move.

We breathe from the moment we are born. When an obstetrician gently slaps a new-born baby's bottom, that baby is encouraged to take his or her first deep lungful of air. The baby's noisy cry of protest as he or she releases that breath is evidence that he or she is alive and well, and there are few parents who don't breathe a deep sigh of relief themselves. But how ironic it is that a baby's first breath should be deep—causing the baby to inhale much more oxygen than his or her tiny body needs and encouraging a damaging pattern of breathing that will be with the child for the rest of his or her life.

This may sound like an unusual concept. If breathing is an involuntary process, how can taking a natural, deep breath be wrong? The answer is quite simple. Breathing is not just involuntary. There are many factors that can cause us to breathe more or less, including stress, panic, emotion and—most important—habit. We can also adjust our rate of breathing, as we do when we hold our breath under water or blow out bursts of air when we exercise.

Most of us breathe incorrectly out of habit, and there are many reasons why this occurs. We are literally trained to overbreathe and have been led to believe that deep breathing is healthy. In times of stress, deliberation, or emotion, we are encouraged to take a deep breath. We have been taught that with every breathing motion we inhale healthy oxygen and exhale a toxic gas called carbon dioxide. Big, deep breaths of fresh air provide us with masses of essential oxygen; exhaling releases the poison. Oxygen is the gas of life, while carbon dioxide is the waste gas.

Therein lies the confusion.

The Carbon Dioxide Myth

Carbon dioxide is not a waste gas. It is one of the most important chemical regulators of the human body, and it is essential for the activity of our hearts, our blood vessels, and our respiratory systems. Carbon dioxide enables oxygen to do its work and, in reality, we need far more carbon dioxide than we do oxygen.

When we overbreathe—that is, breathe more than the physiological norm—we are actually getting less oxygen, not more. This happens because our bodies need to maintain a certain level of carbon dioxide in our blood in order for the red blood cells to release the oxygen we need. When we overbreathe, the balance between carbon dioxide and oxygen in the bloodstream is upset. We may be taking in more oxygen, but we are also breathing out more carbon dioxide, and without the carbon dioxide, our bodies cannot use the oxygen we inhale. We need certain levels of carbon dioxide in our bodies for them to function correctly. When those levels are too low, the chemical bond between oxygen and hemoglobin (which carries oxygen through our blood) increases. In real terms, that means that hemoglobin will not let go of the oxygen it is carrying, which makes it difficult for the cells of our brains, hearts, kidneys, and other organs to get the oxygen they need. As a result, the deeper we breathe, the less oxygen our bodies get.

We now know that all asthmatics overbreathe, and that this rate of overbreathing occurs during asthma attacks. If you stop overbreathing, your asthma will go away. The cause of asthma is hyperventilation, and the way to prevent it is to retrain your breathing.

This book seeks to educate all of us about the way we breathe. It is aimed particularly at asthmatics, parents and carers of asthmatics, and those who suffer from other respiratory conditions. But the fact is that we will all benefit from breathing correctly. We will show that scores of other debilitating conditions, from heart disease to emotional stress, can be relieved and in many cases helped by adopting our new approach to breathing and breath control.

I'm Out of Breath. Out of Breath . . .

It's a common playground cry, as familiar as "It's not fair." But while one child may be panting after competing in and completing a school sports day race or rushing for a catch during a game of football, another child may wheeze and squeeze out the words in desperate pain. For an increasing number of parents, this cry strikes a chord of fear in their hearts. At least one in 10 children in the United Kingdom suffers from asthma, and every week 40 people die from an asthma attack.

It is a tragedy that so many children suffer from asthma and it can be terrible for their parents to watch helplessly as they endure spasms and attacks that could be life-threatening. Asthma reduces quality of life, and whole families can be affected by the needs of one member. Some parents may even feel illogically responsible for the constraints that asthma can place on the lives of their whole family. And despite the fact that asthma is commonly regarded as a childhood affliction, many adults have also been sentenced to a life of fear, one in which a potential attack looms with every deep breath or act of physical exertion.

But it doesn't have to be this way. *I'm out of breath* need never again mean something akin to being out of luck, out of time, or out of funds. Our program is designed to change breathing patterns so that there will never be a need to take great gulps of air after exercise. By retraining breathing and learning correct breath control, gasping for breath becomes unnecessary—for adults, children, asthmatics, and even sports professionals.

Even those of us who find the mildest of exercises—such as walking or carrying home a heavy load from the shops—strenuous will experience an amazing respite from wheezing and heavy breathing. When you have learned to breathe properly and are able to abandon drugs that may have hindered rather than helped you in the past, you will feel better than you could ever have imagined. Your asthmatic child will sleep in peace and grow ever stronger as he or she learns to follow the simple steps that we suggest here.

Healthy breathing should be a birthright, and for many people it is. But for those thousands of people who die each year through asthma and related conditions, breathing became impossible. For the hundreds of thousands of others who have had the quality of their lives destroyed by asthma, breathing is a challenge they face day after day. Most of us don't even think about breathing; asthmatics are forced to think about it constantly.

It's important to remind ourselves that asthma is a killer disease. It is sometimes underestimated or even dismissed because its victims can seem so well most of the time, with no visible bandages, crutches, rashes, temperature, or pain. Yet in the grip of an attack, an asthmatic can feel and indeed be close to death. Such attacks are all the more frightening for the speed at which they occur and their unpredictability.

More and more of us are suffering. Despite, and possibly because of, advances in drug-related treatment, the numbers of sufferers are continuing to soar. Coupled with an outdated and dangerous form of breathing that has become the norm in most Western countries, this epidemic is likely to reach even more frightening proportions.

But we are entering a new age in health care. The god of modern medicine has been proved fallible, and we are, increasingly, looking for alternatives to conventional medical treatment. We are beginning to rely less on a medical system that is overdependent upon drugs and beginning to take some responsibility for our own health. Happily, that means that we are beginning to listen more closely to the messages preserved by older cultures, cultures in which treatment is aimed at uncovering the cause of a condition and actually curing it rather than relying on a barrage of drugs that mask the symptoms and do little at all to effect a cure.

INTRODUCTION

A Drug-Free Life

We do not advocate that all asthmatics should abandon all their drugs and medicines immediately, but we will show here that they can dramatically reduce dosages within five short days. Carefully prescribed steroids may continue to play an essential role in the day-to-day lives of some asthmatics and dosage should only be reduced upon the advice of a general practitioner or a Breath Connection counselor. But for those sufferers who experience milder symptoms, our program will dramatically reduce the need for drugs. And that's not all. Whether you suffer from asthma or a respiratory condition, you will experience better, more peaceful sleep, weight control, emotional balance, professional efficiency, and a sense of well-being that imparts confidence and a renewed zest for life. The threat of other conditions ranging from heart disease to muscular disorders will also be minimized. Even more importantly, you will be given a priceless sense of freedom to live life to the fullest and to reach your individual potential.

Perhaps this sounds too miraculous, too good to be true. Give us five days and we will prove it to you.

Maybe you simply experience occasional panic attacks. If so, you know how debilitating—even terrifying—they can be. Imagine being asthmatic and experiencing the daily dread of something 50 times worse. Imagine attacks that can strike you in professional situations, in public places, or, more frighteningly, at home alone. Panic attacks are close relations of asthma attacks: Both are caused by hyperventilation.

What Is Hyperventilation?

In this book we use the term *hyperventilation* to describe any condition that is caused by overbreathing. *Hyper* means "too much," and *ventilation* refers to lung ventilation, or breathing.

As we discussed earlier, overbreathing, or hyperventilation, starves the body and brain of something it actually needs more than oxygen: carbon dioxide, or CO_2. Carbon dioxide is now known to be essential to every aspect of our good health. Outdated ideas about CO_2's poisonous qualities took root a century ago, around the time when the trees in London's parks were described as the city's lungs. But how would those splendid trees have grown so tall and stood so long without the correct interaction of the carbon dioxide that their trunks and leaves absorbed and the oxygen that was subsequently emitted?

It's time to review old theories and assumptions. Carbon dioxide is now known to be our friend. By breathing more shallowly, lightly, and carefully, we will not lose so much of this essential gas when we exhale. With higher levels of carbon dioxide in our blood, the oxygen will be released more quickly and more steadily from our red blood cells. Whether you suffer from asthma, bronchitis, emphysema, or any other respiratory disorder, you will benefit from correct breathing and your general health will improve dramatically.

Retraining

You may wonder how something as automatic as breathing can be retrained. Isn't the process completely natural? We promise you that the relearning is fast and easy. The deep breathing that many of us were brought up to regard as healthy isn't natural at all. In many parts of the world, people are not taught to breathe deeply, and in those regions the incidence of bronchial disorders is significantly lower than it is here in the West.

Perhaps you are also wondering why reeducating breathing patterns requires a whole book or even attendance at a group session. For most readers, a study of these pages will be sufficient; for others, the benefits of group learning will be more helpful. In either case, it is a matter of positive application, an understanding of the basically sound and scientific principles upon which the Breath Connection program is based, and a little education. A small amount of effort and application will be handsomely rewarded.

Conventional medicine has never really addressed the causes or effects of hyperventilation. Putting it simply, when we hyperventilate, we take in too much air, and we breathe out too much precious carbon dioxide. This means that the body is unable to absorb the small but essential amount of oxygen it needs for all of its interrelated systems to function properly. The Russian professor Konstantin Buteyko discovered that hyperventilation not only causes asthma and other respiratory illnesses, but it lies at the root of nearly 200 other disorders.

We do advise certain dietary changes, and to begin with you will need to concentrate on your breathing exercises for 30 or 40 minutes each day. We also gently recommend that you appraise your general lifestyle, which is ultimately crucial to your overall health and well-being. So, it may take some time and effort over these next days or weeks, but look upon this as the best investment you can possibly make. You'll be investing in yourself—your health and your future. Take a little care, time, and trouble to follow our guidelines and the results and benefits can be immeasurable.

A Revolutionary Approach

The inspiration behind this book and the Breath Connection program of which it forms a part is a distinguished Russian scientist and doctor, Professor Konstantin Buteyko, whose research and work with asthmatics and others with bronchial disorders has only recently been available outside the former Soviet Union. We'll talk more about Professor Buteyko and his pioneering work later in this book and we urge you to study the background of this revolutionary program. Professor Buteyko's discovery is a fascinating one and it is gathering increasing support among both the conventional and complementary health professions.

Here at the Hale Clinic, we have always searched for different approaches—both old and new—to treating the widest range of illnesses and I believe our record speaks for itself. Tried and trusted assumptions about health are never dismissed and we are aware that there is a wealth of advice, gathered across the centuries, that is as applicable today as it was thousands of years ago. We always seek to find complementary solutions to disorders and work in a holistic way with all our patients. Very occasionally, something wonderful and new comes along, such as Professor Buteyko's method—a revolutionary approach to a health problem that challenges one of our most basic instincts: breathing. The Breath Connection program sets out to question the established thinking and to change the way in which we have been taught or trained to breathe. It is an exciting discovery, and the results are unquestionable.

On a personal level, I see the Breath Connection program as one of the most important medical discoveries of the century—and one that will come of age in the next. Although it is our belief that no one system of medicine has all the answers to all the disorders that can strike, we know that Breath Connection has already saved many lives, has transformed the lives of thousands more, and has the potential to help millions.

Just as air cannot be bottled, Breath Connection research cannot be patented. But this is fine with us—we welcome and encourage further research that could do so much for the general health and well-being of millions of people—not just asthmatics. It will be a great day when carefully monitored and assessed collaboration exists—ideally worldwide. For obvious reasons, we cannot expect much encouragement from international pharmaceutical companies who stand to lose from such research, but doubtless they will adapt and we will find our funding elsewhere. Charities could help and so could governments and academic research foundations. Already our work has solicited the supportive interest of some such bodies. It won't happen overnight, but it *will* happen.

Perhaps we are most eager to establish a partnership with the conventional medical establishment. It will be another great day when we work in greater formalized harmony toward the aims of Breath Connection—aims that are, surely, shared by everyone.

Coexistence: Conventional and *Complementary Medicine*

First of all, let me introduce myself. I am Teresa Hale, founder of the Hale Clinic. The clinic was opened in 1988 by the Prince of Wales, whose interest in complementary medicine is well known. My aim was to offer treatments that could integrate conventional and alternative medicine. The strengths of both systems would be called upon to treat patients in a unique setting. Since its inception, the Hale Clinic has explored ideas and treatments from around the globe, and we remain firm in our belief that the most successful kind of health care is one that calls upon the doctrines and methods of a variety of disciplines. No single discipline holds the answer for every patient, and we are able to come up with an individually tailored treatment plan for all types of patients, based on the very best of leading therapeutic systems around the world. As a result, the clinic has become a sort of United Nations for complementary medicine and the fact that we continue to grow suggests that we have simply addressed a need that was waiting to be met. The clinic is based in central London, but we hold courses all over the United Kingdom. We are strong believers in the power of self-help, so no readers should feel disadvantaged if they are not within easy reach of us. We see health as a personal journey for the individual, and it is important to find the right path for each of our patients. With over 100 practitioners offering a broad range of conventional and holistic treatments, we are well placed to meet specific needs.

A few years ago, I was intrigued by the enthusiasm of a fellow professional who had heard about Professor Konstantin Buteyko's extraordinary work with asthmatic patients in the former Soviet Union. There wasn't much to read at that stage, but I was impressed by his results and managed to speak to some people who had taken part in his courses. Their responses ranged from being hugely enthusiastic to positively evangelical. From them and from his preliminary research I learned about his Breath Control methods and resolved to delve further, holding a course at the Hale Clinic based on his work. I was startled by the improvements observed in both the attitude and the health of asthmatics.

It wasn't just the fact that bronchial problems had been dramatically diminished, or even the fact that all of the patients who visited the clinic had either abandoned previous medication entirely or had greatly reduced their need for it. What also caught my attention were the other, unexpected benefits to the treatment. Peoples' appetites had become balanced and stabilized so that even the very overweight were shedding pounds while dangerously underweight patients had recovered an interest in the right kinds of food and were building up strength. Balanced breathing had led to balanced eating. There also seemed to be an awakening of confidence and a general increase in energy as well as relief from distressing sleep patterns and the daytime fears and discomfort that most asthmatics endure.

I was amused to learn that English patients who received treatment with Professor Buteyko's method in Russia had enjoyed little of the cozy bedside manner that we prize so much in Britain. The system had been explained to them, they were told to follow the guidelines and expected to get on with it. Oddly, this brusque attitude rather impressed the English patients who reasoned, correctly, that no clinic attempting to peddle a dubious treatment would treat the patients with so little pampering. I became more and more intrigued, making it my business to learn as much as possible about Buteyko's methods.

I learned that although his findings are now treated with the greatest respect in Russia, this wasn't always the case. For years, his work had been undervalued, and certainly, before the rapprochement between East and West, there was little interest in his work from doctors outside the Soviet Union. Unwittingly, my interest in his work has helped to bring a revolutionary and truly lifesaving technique to the West.

I, too, was full of enthusiasm when I found myself talking about the method to an American journalist, after speaking to a group of businesswomen at a dinner in London. She showed more than a polite interest and suggested that I meet her agent, Al Lowman, when I was next in New York. Al, she said, had such severe asthma that his doctor had recommended a lung operation that would cost in the region of $90,000. When I met him soon afterward, I did not promise that the clinic could cure his asthma but I was pretty sure that we could enable him to reduce his medication, to suffer far fewer attacks, and to walk upstairs or along a corridor without gasping for breath every few steps.

Although by nature skeptical, Al was impressed by my absolute confidence and general approach. Soon afterward, he braved a flight to London—during which he endured a near-fatal asthma attack—to visit us at the clinic and to learn about the incredibly simple shallow-breathing techniques that have spared the lives of thousands of asthmatics and others suffering from related illnesses. Al was adamant that I should write this book. It would have been impossible for him to return to The Hale Clinic for follow-up treatments, and he was well aware that few of the 6,000 Americans who die from asthma every year could do so either. He was right. This book is of real value both to those who suffer as severely as Al does and to the scores of thousands more who have milder but nonetheless distressing symptoms.

I decided to stress how a revised diet and exercise regime can help many people and to point out the importance of educating people to understand the nature of the asthma and its severity. By coincidence, as I was in the early stages of planning this book, there was an outstanding BBC1 TV documentary, produced by Norman Stone, about the effectiveness of Professor Buteyko's techniques. It raised questions about why the established medical profession seemed to be dismissive. This cutting-edge program closely reflected my own interest in the area. A phenomenal 7 million people watched the show and the BBC was inundated with requests for further information about Professor Buteyko's method.

I was more determined than ever to spread the word about the Buteyko principles. It also inspired me to do all I could to ensure that Breath Connection classes and workshops were accessible to people in every major city in the United Kingdom. This book will be the perfect complement to those classes, and if you are, for whatever reason, unable to attend the classes, it will provide the basic grounding you need to understand the principles behind this unique treatment. This book sets out to relieve you, or anyone you care for, from the shackles of asthma and other bronchial or respiratory illnesses for life.

Like me, Norman Stone was alarmed to discover that a killer disease such as asthma had no cure. Conventional medicine addresses the symptoms and eases the suffering, but it does nothing to treat or uncover the root cause. In the program, he featured three seriously ill asthmatics who followed a five-day course. After that short period, all were well on their way to leading normal lives again. People whose lives were seriously restricted were enjoying sport; an anorexic demanded food. Norman Stone also drew attention to the fact that no medical research establishments in Britain were set up to investigate this horrifying disease. This is, perhaps, a sad reflection of our approach to the condition. Despite the fact that it kills thousands each year, asthma is still not receiving the attention that it deserves.

Indeed, despite his landmark successes, Professor Buteyko's ideas were largely ignored if not actually impeded in Russia for nearly 40 years. Better late than never, however, for the millions worldwide who endure this underestimated and almost invisible disorder.

It is extraordinary to think that work begun by a young Russian doctor would result in over 45 years of practical and scientific research into the major causes of over 200 medical conditions currently considered to be incurable by conventional medicine. The simplicity of Buteyko's theories— namely, that asthma is caused by hyperventilation—should not lead anyone to underestimate the depth, extent, and complexity of the scientific research that led to this momentous discovery. His studies are a cause for celebration for anyone who stands to benefit from them.

In the past, Professor Buteyko expressed his hope that freer societies would provide people with the right to choose their medical treatment without constraint. The society in which he lived and practiced did not allow patients the luxury of choice, and his 40-year battle during the pioneering stages of his work led him to the conclusion that people must be able, and encouraged, to choose the treatment system that is right for them and their individual conditions. Most importantly, treatment should be readily available to all who need it. Let us hope that in Britain, the United States, and other Western countries, this vision will become a reality. Bodies such as the National Health Service in the United Kingdom need to recognize the importance of the Breath

Connection program and to make its benefits freely available to every one of the huge population of asthma sufferers.

Our Promises

We promise to utilize everything that modern science, communication, and technology can offer, as well as our own tried and tested methods, to help improve every aspect of the quality of your life. We promise to respect you as an individual and to offer support at every level. These are not shallow or hollow promises. Even if you follow the program for only five days, there has to be effort and commitment on your part—particularly if you decide to keep going for weeks, or even months. It is never easy to break a habit or to learn a new skill, and it's only human to consider lapsing from time to time. We believe that the results that can be achieved by practicing the program for just a short time each day, over five days, will encourage you to keep going. Soon, the Breath Connection program will become second nature, and you will continue to reap the benefits.

In the meantime, here is an introduction for everyone who wants to breathe more easily and to be freed and released from the unnecessary constraints of any one of a host of health conditions. Whether you suffer from antisocial snoring or life-threatening asthma, this book addresses no more than the breath of life—*and no less.*

1

Into the Next Century

Breathing is our first affirmation when we enter the world. Our last breath signals our departure. Death is an experience beyond human understanding, and our ways of approaching it range between calm and panic. Personal spiritual beliefs may well play a major part in the way we see death, but they are far beyond the remit of this book. What we are concerned about is life, and our certain belief that your earthly life can be enhanced long into the next century by the ideas we embrace.

For those of you who are depressed or discouraged by your asthma, or another health condition, it is worth remembering that huge advances have been made in medicine in the twentieth century. So far, we have focused on the fact that asthma is underestimated and that we are no nearer to a cure than we were decades ago. But in all fields, not just medicine, the daily quality of our lives has improved dramatically, and there is no reason to suppose that this exponential improvement in our general comfort and well-being will not continue in this lifetime. Think about the advances and improvements in the quality of our lives and leisure time or the disappearance of such diseases as polio and small pox, which were regarded as common only a few decades ago. Our age has seen the emergence of some new, or newly identified, illnesses, such as AIDS and CJD (Creutzfeldt-Jakob disease), but on the basis of past successes, aren't we right to believe that these can be managed and conquered just as the killer diseases were in the past?

Many of us have grown up in the age of huge scientific advance and may simply take these wonders in our stride. We live in an amazing time, and now, more than ever, we can use the significant scientific discoveries and the wealth of information from around the world for our own personal benefit. We are relearning about our bodies and their miraculous ability to respond to treatment of all kinds.

We should welcome our new century with confidence. We have the benefit of a rich past to call upon, and we can open our eyes to the new discoveries of the future.

Even the most fundamental aspects of our lives are now being given attention. It is, perhaps, surprising that breath and breathing—the most basic and necessary element of our daily lives—have received so little attention. Considering the number of extensive studies undertaken on nutrition and exercise, breathing has been the subject of very little medical research. Firm in the belief that all treatment should be holistic, we at the Hale Clinic believe that research into all of the body's functions and systems is equally important and necessarily interlinked.

Asthma has, until recently, remained a mystery. More cases were reported in the former West Germany, where access to sophisticated medicines and treatment were readily available, than in the less technically advanced and highly polluted East. In Britain, asthma is as common in the cleanest parts of the countryside as it is in London. While pollution may exacerbate the condition in asthmatics, we now know that it is not the cause. This is where the Breath

Connection program has a great deal to offer. After decades of research, Professor Buteyko has finally uncovered the cause of asthma. We still have a great deal to learn about this life-threatening condition, but the Breath Connection program has made extraordinary strides in both the understanding and educational training for asthma. We can offer much more than relief for your respiratory problems. Using a unique preventative health program, we now have the means by which to give our children the basis of sound health for life. And all of us can experience better health as a result of the training offered through the program.

This Is What We Promise

The Breath Connection program requires no medication, no special equipment or technology, and simply aims to reeducate people about how to breathe in a balanced, healthier way. Apart from helping you to overcome a debilitating illness and to enhance your health generally, we hope that this book will encourage further research into the importance and value of carbon dioxide. In Appendix B, we discuss a host of other illnesses that have responded to the Breath Connection program. We hope this book will draw attention to these ailments and inspire more studies and research. All doctors, nurses, physiotherapists, and other hospital professionals need to learn the Breath Connection methods as part of their training. They can be utilized alongside the best of the current conventional and complementary techniques and offer the first real hope of a breakthrough in the treatment of asthma, and a host of other conditions, to date.

An asthmatic who has contracted pneumonia could, for example, be treated with antibiotics in the first instance, and then taught Breath Connection so that his or her immune system is strengthened and the risk of recurring illness lessened. Heart surgery could, for many patients, be avoided if a hospital specialist had worked with a Breath Connection practitioner. I also hope to see many practitioners in the complementary fields—such as acupuncturists, homeopaths, and chiropractors—utilizing the tool to help their patients. As a remedy for common, but nonetheless distressing, conditions such as colds, flu, sinusitis, and sore throats, Breath Connection has a wide range of uses, the first and foremost being an ability to encourage the immune system in a way that antibiotics will never do. The British government has acknowledged the futility of prescribing antibiotics for viral conditions that simply do not respond to them and has urged doctors to be more wary in prescribing them, to prevent a surge of superbugs that are resistant to antibiotics. By using the Breath Connection program, the need for antibiotics is diminished, and because it works to boost immunity, the overall health of the population will improve.

In the business community, I see Breath Connection being used to enhance concentration and performance. Businesspeople in all walks of life would experience greater energy and could function well with less sleep, something that may become an increasing necessity in our competitive world. Good health is essential if we are to cope with stress in the workplace, and Breath Connection offers fast stress relief, quite apart from its other benefits. The additional effects of this would be a reduction in absenteeism, as well as increased alertness and productivity. In the future, employees may be entitled to sue their employers for conditions caused by stress in the workplace, so it makes sense that employers should endeavor to prevent stress before it becomes a serious problem. By supplying basic facilities, such as a quiet room and regular breaks for staff to perform Breath Connection exercises at work, employers would reap the benefits of a healthier, more productive workforce.

Schools also need to consider the implications of the Breath Connection program. It is, in particular, helpful for hyperactive children, as well as those with attention deficit disorders, allergies, and a range of respiratory conditions. Children will have a better ability to focus on the job at hand and will learn more quickly and efficiently. If the exercises are learned at an early age, children will undoubtedly achieve better results at school, as well as experience a dramatic decline in illnesses. If mothers practice breath control while pregnant, more oxygen will reach their babies' bodies and brains, giving them a good start in life.

Adopting the Breath Connection program on a broad scale across nations would have ramifications for everyone. Governments would save vast amounts of money on unnecessary treatments. Premiums for private medical insurance should, logically, be reduced for the same reasons. In the 1998 QED program documenting Professor Buteyko's work, Dr. Gerald Spence said that the annual cost of drugs per annum, for each asthmatic patient, fell by two-thirds once Professor Buteyko's method had been employed. Breath Connection could save Britain's strained National Health Service about £330 million every year. In the United States, where medical care is often dictated by the level of health insurance and health maintenance policies, this is even more significant.

And costs will be reduced for a whole host of other ailments as well. For example, we now know that impotence is largely caused by vascular problems, and Breath Connection is a far cheaper alternative to Viagra. Better circulation, as a result of the program, ensures that blood reaches the penis and both achieves and sustains an erection.

International sportsmen and -women, such as the 1994 Australian football team, have found that Breath Connection enhanced their stamina and performance. The techniques can reduce symptoms of high physical stress, such as headaches, blocked noses and fevers, psychological pressures, and the problems experienced while training and competing in unfamiliar climatic conditions. Performance at the highest level can be enhanced by the athlete's increased ability to cope with pressures of every kind. Even at local park kick-around level, Breath Connection can help to improve performance and increase enjoyment.

Even more crucial for the Western world is the fact that Breath Connection enables people to reach their natural weight. Reconditioned breathing speeds up the metabolism and balances the hormonal system. Carbon dioxide influences the function and performance of the pancreas, which controls our blood sugar, our metabolism, and, through that, our weight. In a relatively short time, the overweight can shed pounds and experience a reduced appetite, while the underweight will begin to eat healthily again. We are not in the beauty business, but there is no question that overweight and underweight can lead to health problems. We want to see a normalization of our patients' weight, and we have observed startling changes in eating habits and weight as a result of the Breath Connection program.

The Will to Be Well

As you can see, Breath Connection offers a simple program to rebalance the whole body and to improve the quality of every area of your lives. The success of the program depends on you, and your willingness to set aside a little time for just a few days. If your problems are more severe, you may need to invest a little more time, but we can promise that you will begin to see encouraging results in as little as five days. You must also resolve to make a few dietary and lifestyle changes if you want the program to fulfill its promise of changing your life for the better—forever.

Each of us has to decide how much we want to make changes—how much regeneration we want to see, and how willing we are to accept degeneration in our bodies. It goes without saying that the majority of us do want to reach our own full potential, but there are some of us—with our own complex psychological reasons, which we will discuss later—who cling to the familiarity and comfort of illness. Nothing worth achieving comes easily, and to achieve the best, you have to be prepared to give your best. Always remember that you are investing in yourself and your future health. While the majority of us may not be ill in the accepted medical sense, chances are that we are not functioning at our full potential. It is often the case that we don't realize that we did feel unwell until we experience the full benefits of optimum health and well-being. Whether or not you have a recognized illness to confront, you can be helped by the Breath Connection program.

I have a term for certain people who seem to be functioning well, with little effort: *the vertically ill*. These people may be standing up straight and coping on a day-to-day level, but beneath the surface, their body systems are working double shifts to keep them that way. The body does not have unlimited resources, and when it is forced to work hard to maintain an equilibrium, there will, eventually, come a time when it is unable to continue. All of us can benefit from Breath Connection, whatever our age or level of health and fitness. In fact, people who do not suffer from an obvious illness will find the program remarkably easy to adopt, and it takes no time at all to get into the habit of practicing the Breath Connection exercises almost anywhere. With the exercises under your belt, and a few dietary and lifestyle changes, you will feel stronger and more energized in every possible way. By achieving your own individual potential, all aspects of your life will be changed: You will sleep better, work more efficiently, look great, and enjoy life more fully. You don't need to spend money on special equipment, gyms, or extra treatments—the improvements will be evident through breathing alone.

A simple Control Pause will tell you if you stand to benefit from Breath Connection. If you can't hold your breath out comfortably for 45 seconds, there is a strong chance that you will experience illness later in life. Don't put something as vital as your health on hold. That back burner may be slow, but it allows things to simmer. . . .

If you do suffer from a life-threatening illness, such as emphysema, you need to ask yourself if you want to be dependent upon drugs for the rest of your life, without any guarantee that they will improve its quality. Or would you prefer to control the illness our way, alleviating its symptoms and allowing you to start participating in your life again. It's up to you. At the very least, you stand to gain a vastly improved stake in the control of your life. In a later chapter, we will show that you don't have to continue down the drugs route and that making changes really is possible.

If you can find the time to spend half an hour leafing through a magazine or polishing the kitchen floor, you can find the time for Breath Connection. Think about your retirement and any money you may be paying into a pension fund. How wasteful it will prove to be if you aren't well enough to enjoy the last third of your life. Think about your children. You want to be healthy enough to watch them grow up, and, even more importantly, you want to watch them do well in life. By investing the time and energy now, your whole family can benefit in the years to come. It's all time that can be clawed back in other forms. For example, the Breath Connection program encourages deeper, more restful sleep, and you'll find that you need far less of it. You can use part of the time you have gained to practice a program that will affect your whole life.

Many of the treatments we now practice, such as herbalism, ayurveda, and acupuncture, are, in fact, based on age-old wisdom. They are now becoming accepted in the conventional medical system and have encouraged a new holistic view of treatment. It is rare when something recent and modern, not involving drugs, comes along. Professor Buteyko's findings are just that—a real breakthrough in the history of medicine based on modern research and a recent discovery. It is my dearest wish that the Buteyko principles will become accepted in the same way that ancient wisdom has experienced a renaissance. We are all working toward the same goal, that of relieving unnecessary pain and suffering, and we need to have the vision to embrace discoveries, both new and old, with equal fervor.

There is a great deal of evidence that the act of helping oneself can encourage positive health, and Professor Buteyko's methods are based on self-help. We live in an age when health is becoming a priority, and more and more of us are taking steps to ensure that we are getting the best, and doing the best we can, for optimum health and well-being. Public demand encourages change. Supermarkets now stock a wide range of organic foods because the public insisted they wanted them. Herbs and homeopathic remedies are available at most pharmacies, when only five years ago they were considered by many to be distinctly alternative. If the same interest and enthusiasm is shown for the Breath Connection program, the demand will encourage the changes we want to see in our health services, and the way we address health in general.

Explain what you want to your doctor. With luck he or she will be sympathetic and helpful. The results speak for themselves, and no doctor can fail to be interested in something that provides genuine relief from ill health of any description. We can only hope that conventional medicine will see the light and begin to offer this treatment alongside, or in place of, drugs. In the meantime, take heart from the guidance we offer here and show, by shining example, that you, as the owner of your body, know best.

The Expansion of Health

We often see the phrase *optimal health* in books and articles. It sounds like a vague term, even if it is a laudable aim. The importance of ginger tea, or broccoli, food combining, special exercises, and even cider vinegar have all been attributed with the power to provide optimal health. So many regimes promise instant perfection, and most of us are, of course, healthily skeptical. There is no such thing as perfection, but what you are aiming for is what is the best for you. *Optimum* or *optimal health* means achieving the best health you possibly can, for you as an individual. We don't promise perfection. We offer a result in five days which acts as a foundation to good health, a springboard from which you can only get better.

The teachers of ancient systems such as acupuncture and

the Indian system of life, ayurveda, considered good health to be an equilibrium within the body. Massages, needles, and herbs were employed to balance energy through meridians or channels that run through our bodies. Yoga, T'ai chi, and Qi Gong programs were adopted to encourage equilibrium, and those same disciplines are used today with equally good results. Breath Connection follows these same principles. We believe that good health can be achieved and maintained through correct breathing. When the body has a correct balance of oxygen and carbon dioxide, the right environment is created for the expansion of our health. You will see how balanced breathing not only prevents disease, but expands our capacity for good health.

In the West, the average life span is 78 years. This may sound like a long time until we consider the longevity of people living in remote enclaves of the Himalayas or the Andes. In these regions, some people are known to live for 120 or even 150 years without enduring ill health or degenerative disease as they grow older. So, the possibility of expanding not only health but life span clearly exists. The long life that is common to these regions is full and pain-free. At Breath Connection, we believe we know how to establish similar patterns that will work here in the West.

We have spent a great deal of time, energy, and financial resources effectively fire fighting. We have lost the knack of preventing the fire in the first place. It can never be repeated too often that prevention is better than cure. Health expansion begins with monitoring your daily progress by checking your pulse and measuring your breathing rate with a daily series of Control Pauses (see page 48). Early improvements in the way you look, feel, and sleep will encourage you to continue with the program until every vital system in your body is primed to last long beyond that 78-year mark.

Reading and understanding the principles that underpin this book are excellent ways to begin your journey on the road to a long, fulfilling life. You will experience improved mental and physical function for as long as you live. As we have stressed earlier, you can achieve a great deal by yourself. With the help of a Breath Connection course or workshop, you can go even further. Classes are now held in cities across the United Kingdom and the United States, and many people find it easier to retrain their breathing under the supervision of one of our counselors. If you think you need extra coaching, try the classes. Or, put your time and energy into learning the methods described in this book for a lifetime of better health. You may wish to extend your life well into your second century, enjoying children, grandchildren, and even great-grandchildren, and for this you may need some extra help. It's a little like playing tennis or any other sport. If you want to enjoy your game, you can do so by practicing on your own and following simple guidelines. However, if you want to get to Wimbledon, or even aspire to being a local champion, you need a first-rate coach and you need to begin work as soon as possible. Whatever your goals, we think you will be startled and delighted by the results you will achieve with Breath Connection. Anyone can embark on this journey of life expansion, and you can improve the quality and depth of your life as well as living much, much longer.

This journey is for everyone, from pregnant mothers wishing to give the best possible start to their unborn babies, to the elderly; from children of all ages to people in their middle ages. Whether you are well or have a history of frailty, you will experience positive change with this program.

Regeneration

As soon as you begin the Breath Connection program, your digestive system starts to function more efficiently. Sluggish metabolisms are given a kick-start, and food is more swiftly converted to energy. Nutrients are more easily absorbed by the body, and toxins are more easily excreted. Food cravings will reduce as the pancreas functions correctly, and the pH balance of your body will be corrected, leading to improved resistance to food allergies and a stronger immune system.

The body's elimination system will also start to function better. This is not merely bowel function, but the pores and sweat glands that are crucial for the excretion of toxins. We need to absorb and extract goodness from food while losing, as quickly as possible, any toxic residues. Much of our food is sprayed with pesticides and fertilizers, and then processed. Our bodies need to take what nutrition our food has to offer, and then excrete the harmful additives and chemicals before damage can take place.

We also need to start thinking about hygiene. Naturally, you wash daily and launder your clothes regularly. Your house may be immaculate, especially your kitchen. You need to apply the same care to your body that you do to your home. If you don't flush out toxic waste from your body, it would be just as damaging, or offensive, as not flushing your toilet for several days, or allowing old food to molder in a filthy refrigerator. Give your liver, kidneys, and bowels a helping hand by breathing correctly so that they function well.

To ensure that your heart is strong enough to take you through a long life, you need to look after your cardiovascular system. With Breath Connection, circulation will improve, and the danger of high blood pressure, palpitations, and any form of collapse will be reduced. Respect the complex network of your hormonal system. It's not just the thyroid gland that ensures the healthy working of your endocrine system. The pineal gland, the pituitary, and the thymus are all connected and important. They in turn affect the pancreas, itself an important endocrine gland, which affects other parts of the body. Breath Connection is holistic, which means that it is aimed at treating all of you, not just one single part.

The nervous system also needs to be well-tuned to cope with the inevitable pressures of life. Good health and strength can make any pressure easier to bear, but when all systems are working at their peak level, problems are more quickly and efficiently dealt with. We can't promise you a life without anxiety or stress, but we can promise you a better way of dealing with the challenges. Once you are eating properly, breathing correctly, and sleeping well, you are far better placed to cope. Extra blood reaching the brain through correct breathing will make it easier to concentrate upon and solve intellectual dilemmas and to deal with emotional ones as well. The calm and peaceful sleep that you will experience increases this effect.

Perhaps you don't want to live until you are 120; perhaps your aim is to experience good health and well-being in the here and now. The process can begin at any age. We want to help you to empower yourself.

It begins with a simple, single breath.

2

Overbreathing

*And what it is to cease breathing but to free the breath
from its restless tides, that it may rise and expand and seek
God unencumbered?*

Kahlil Gibran, *The Prophet*

What does the word *hyperventilation* mean to you? For
some, it may mean rapid, shallow gasps and for others fast,
deep gulps. Almost everyone will conjure up a picture of
someone panting, red-faced and distressed, possibly after
overstrenuous exercise or during an asthma attack. Medical
dictionaries usually define it as "abnormally rapid deep
breathing."

By Professor Buteyko's definition, *hyperventilation* is
what happens when someone habitually breathes more than
four to six liters of air into their lungs every minute. This
quantity of air is the correct amount for all adults and children—but obviously varies between three and six liters
depending on whether you are a child or a large man—and
leads to very quiet, gentle, and almost undetectable breathing, rather like that of a sleeping baby. Nine out of 10 of us,
however, overbreathe. We have become so accustomed to
breathing deeply that we regularly lose vital carbon dioxide
when we exhale.

Try the Control Pause test on page 48. This simple test is
designed to assess your risk of suffering from hyperventila-
tion-related diseases.

Studies have shown that asthmatics inhale anything between four and eight times the amount of air they need for optimum health, often breathing through the mouth, rather than the nose. This type of overbreathing, or hyperventilation, puts tremendous strain on our body systems, such as the digestive, hormonal, circulation, cardiovascular, and elimination systems. This dysfunctional breathing can be corrected by the Breath Connection program.

Deep Breathing Test

This quick test will help to show you how harmful deep breathing can be. Do not try it if you are a severe asthmatic or epileptic.

Breathe rapidly through your mouth, as if you have been taking part in a fast run. Try to maintain this for several minutes. Have a pencil and paper on hand and make a note of how quickly you experience any of the following symptoms:

- Dizziness
- Chest pains
- Palpitations
- Blocked nose
- Coughing
- Feeling faint
- Headache

These effects will have occurred because your physiological systems have been starved of carbon dioxide.

Now begin to breathe slowly and shallowly through your nose. We call this type of breathing *balanced breathing*, in which the equilibrium between levels of oxygen and carbon dioxide in the respiratory system is maintained. See how quickly the symptoms of overbreathing are reversed.

We should stress that our definitions of deep and shallow breathing relate to the amount of air that is inhaled and we're often asked to explain why in many yogic exercises people are, conversely, encouraged to take deep breaths. It's not actually so very different. When practicing yoga, you are encouraged to breathe very slowly, and through the nose. You do not hyperventilate because the amount of air you take in is restricted. Other techniques, such as rebirthing,

Yogic breathing

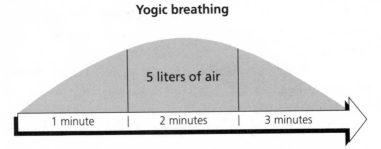

5 liters of air breathed over 3 minutes.

Asthmatic breathing

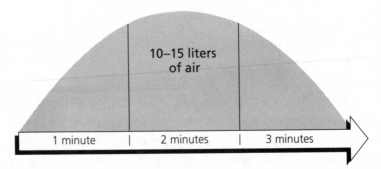

10–15 liters of air breathed over 3 minutes.

34

encourage shallow, rapid breathing, called *panting*. We do not feel that this is a healthy way to breathe.

Why Orthodox Modern Medicine Can't Cure Asthma and Emphysema

Every idea in this book is underpinned by the strongest belief in a holistic approach to health. All of our advice must be considered alongside diet, sleeping, and exercise habits—your lifestyle in general. These are all important aspects of your health, and addressing only one tiny part will not have the same effect as broadscale measures that take into consideration all of the factors that make you and your lifestyle individual. In later chapters, we address other essential aspects of our holistic approach. Here, however, we offer some very specific information and answers to what has been one of the most crucial health challenges of our age.

Asthma and emphysema are defense mechanisms against hyperventilation, created by the body to counter a loss of carbon dioxide. This mechanism induces spasms of the bronchotubes, creating inflammation and excess mucus or a reduced lung capacity. Any attempt to treat asthma or emphysema without dealing with hyperventilation as the underlying cause is doomed to fail. Dealing with hyperventilation, or overbreathing, is the central tenet of the Breath Connection program.

Many therapies and some drugs, including the use of nebulizers, can provide some temporary relief, but artificially suppressing what is actually the body's natural defense mechanism will further increase hyperventilation and cause the body to implement some other line of defense. By suppressing your asthma, you could develop emphysema, pulmonary fibrosis, heart disease, diabetes, epilepsy, or cancer in its place because your body still has to find some means of preventing you from hyperventilating and expelling too much carbon dioxide. Further, the more often you resort to using a bronchodilator or taking steroids, the more you will come to depend on them. Asthma is not cured by modern medical treatments, its symptoms are merely suppressed. The cause still remains and if we continually ignore our body's message that something is wrong, the condition will become much, much worse.

Many asthmatics start with the occasional puff on an inhaler for quick relief, but soon depend on a battery of nebulizers and steroids. Some may need hospital treatment. The reason for this dependency and the overall degeneration of the condition is solely because doctors have been treating symptoms rather than the disease itself.

The conventional treatment for asthma and emphysema is drugs or physiotherapy—both of which actually cause hyperventilation. This is akin to treating an alcoholic with vodka or a diabetic with sugar. This practice is not to be confused with the considered homeopathic principle of treating like with like.

The Respiratory System

The Lungs
The right lung has three lobes and the left two, each comprising numerous lobules bound by connective tissue. Within each of them is a group of air chambers bearing small pouches called *alveoli*.

During inhalation, air passes through the windpipe into the main airways attached to each lung. The oxygen in the air dissolves into the alveoli and is diffused through these cells and through capillary walls into blood plasma. From the plasma, the oxygen molecules combine with hemoglobin in the red blood cells to form oxyhemoglobin. This process allows the blood to carry approximately 70 times more oxygen than it would normally. Once this blood reaches the body cells where oxygen in required, its oxygen load is released. The trigger for this release is carbon dioxide which, converted to carbonic acid, allows it to be freed. When there is insufficient CO_2 due to overbreathing, the amount of oxygen available to the brain, heart, kidneys, and every other organ in the body is restricted. As a result, essential functions are impaired. Oxygen starvation excites the breathing center of the brain and thus the desire to hyperventilate increases.

Oxygen and carbon dioxide are, thus, partners and not enemies within our system. Carbon dioxide also regulates the body's acid/alkaline balance (also called pH), which is essential for a healthy immune system.

Asthma attack

Normal breathing

Asthmatic's breathing

Bronchotubes open
Normal level of CO_2 and O_2

Broncho restriction
Less than normal level of
CO_2 and O_2

The illustration on page 37 is a simplified representation of what happens to the bronchotubes during an asthma attack. The fairly straight line (*top left*) represents shallow breathing, or normal breathing. Both oxygen and carbon dioxide can move through the clear bronchotubes. To the right you can see the jerky depths and peaks of asthmatic breathing and the bronchial restriction caused by inhaling and exhaling too deeply. The asthmatic is losing too much CO_2 so the bronchotubes have narrowed as the body fights to retain the carbon dioxide which is essential for so many of its functions.

The Causes of Overbreathing and Hyperventilation

Even before we are born we may be affected by the deep-breathing exercises that our pregnant mothers followed so trustingly. Then we were probably encouraged to announce our safe arrival with an outraged scream followed by a deep breath. Later, at school and beyond, we were encouraged to take deep breaths if we felt faint, giddy, or exhausted after strenuous exercise.

Apart from being taught to deep breathe, we have also created a scenario where our oxygen needs are higher, which encourages us instinctively to overbreathe, or to breathe more deeply in a misguided attempt to satisfy our oxygen needs.

Take, for example, our eating habits. A high-protein diet—until quite recently regarded as healthy and desirable—places severe strain on many of our bodies' systems and creates a pattern of overbreathing. The amount of oxygen energy needed to digest a protein meal, whether it is made up of vegetable or animal proteins, is similar to the amount needed for a brisk walk. More information about diet and nutrition follows in a later section of this book where we describe the foods that will help you not to overbreathe.

Sleeping correctly is enormously important, and very little advice has been given about the correct way to sleep. Many of us have a tendency to sleep on our backs, which causes breathing to deepen. Sleeping with our mouths open compounds the problem. Most epileptic fits, strokes, and paralysis happen at the end of a long sleeping period when the sleeper is about to waken. It is no coincidence that these occur after a long period of deep breathing.

Meditation and controlled relaxation encourage shallow breathing. Stress and emotional pressure tends to make breathing heavier. Try to avoid stressful situations and emotional confrontations late at night, which can cause breathing to deepen. Restful, peaceful sleep relies on calm, shallow breathing. Overheated, polluted, and confined spaces at night should also be avoided. Arrange your pillows to the left side to help prop you into a correct position (see pages 52–53). Your breathing will be shallower throughout the night as a result. Even Professor Buteyko has no scientific explanation for this phenomenon, but he has observed, in thousands of cases, that it works.

One technique we recommend is to tape your mouth up at night, thus ensuring that you breathe through your nose. This can be particularly effective for children (see Chapter 10) and is not as drastic as it may sound. There is a special tape that is light and painless to remove and apply. We suggest you use this tape until you have learned to breathe through your nose.

If we ensure that we get plenty of carbon dioxide at night, hyperventilation, anxiety, insomnia, and, quite possibly, irritability, stress, and panic attacks will decrease.

The Link Between Carbon Dioxide Starvation and Disease

By now we know about the importance of the natural collaboration between oxygen and carbon dioxide and how their partnership helps our bodies to function at full strength every day. And we know that hyperventilation deprives us of the benefits of that partnership. What follows is a short list of some of the many roles carbon dioxide plays in helping us to maintain a healthy, balanced body:

- Oxygenation of vital tissues and organs.
- Maintenance of the acid-alkali (pH) balance necessary for a strong, healthy immune system, without which we are prone to allergies and recurrent infection.
- Smooth muscle dilation, which helps to prevent the sort of spasms which lead to migraine as well as asthma attacks. Such spasms also narrow the arterial vessels, causing varicose veins and hemorrhoids. A spasm is the body's way of preventing the loss of too much CO_2 and is yet another example of the body's defense mechanism against overbreathing.
- Regulation of nervous system activity which prevents the body from going into an unnecessary "fight or flight" mode that can exacerbate stress levels.
- Regulation of a healthy cardiovascular system without which we can suffer from abnormal blood pressure, hypertension, angina, chest pains, and strokes.
- Maintenance of a healthy digestive system, particularly the level of gastric juices needed for efficient breakdown of ingested foods.
- The natural elimination of toxic substances.

As you can see, the Breath Connection program is not only for asthmatics or people suffering from respiratory problems. Dealing with the devil of hyperventilation provides massive benefits for everyone. Oxygen is not the only gas of life. We need carbon dioxide, too. We need to change a previously unchallenged way of thinking and accept that the demon is not a toxic gas, but a way of breathing.

At The Hale Clinic, we are convinced that, despite extraordinary success with our program for those with asthma and other related disorders, the crucially important role of carbon dioxide in holistic health has only just begun to be explored.

These are the facts about hyperventilation, which could remain an invisible killer well into the twenty-first century:

• Up to 90 percent of people in the developed world suffer from illnesses caused by hyperventilation.

• The root cause of so many of these illnesses—ranging from asthma to chronic fatigue—is not yet recognized by orthodox medicine as being hyperventilation. Conventional medicine can greatly alleviate symptoms of these and other illnesses, but it has been unable to reach any firm conclusions about the causes.

• Doctors don't study hyperventilation at medical school and are, therefore, unaware of its very real dangers.

• Most doctors are unable to recognize, diagnose, or treat hyperventilation except in its most acute form.

• Even those few doctors who treat hyperventilation do not do so very effectively.

• Modern medicine uses drugs and deep-breathing exercises to treat hyperventilation, treatments which may relieve symptoms in the short term, but which aggravate the condition in the long term.

- Modern medical theory has not established, nor attempted to establish, the link between hyperventilation and respiratory diseases. Asthma and other respiratory diseases are blamed on a host of unrelated causes and triggers, including the environment, stress, smoking, cats, dogs, cut grass, red wine, butter, salt, sugar, cholesterol, calories, *Candida*, the weather, flu, colds, and dust mites. Some of these may indeed be triggers for some people, but they are not the cause of asthma or any other respiratory disease. Blaming these triggers for asthma is akin to blaming rats for the Black Death plague of the fourteenth century. Certainly the rats transported the bacilli that spread the plague but they didn't create the plague or the disease itself.

- The common ignorance of the physiology of breathing has lead to a situation where the killer phrase *take a deep breath* has become the most popular—and dangerous—advice offered in stress management. This advice is offered to combat panic attacks, anxiety, asthma, and emphysema within fitness classes, schools, hospitals, and sporting establishments.

- More and more people, including—tragically—children, breathe through their mouths. Yet doctors and teachers rarely offer advice against this fast track to hyperventilation. A general national awareness of the importance of breathing through our noses would make a massive difference to public health. Most asthmatics and emphysemics have been advised to deep breathe, little realizing this will deprive them of oxygen rather than supply it.

- Pregnant mothers are taught to deep breathe during labor. If a woman hyperventilates during pregnancy there is a danger that her child will be affected by her hyperventilation habits while it is in the womb and certainly when it is born.

• Various deep-breathing techniques and exercises, including lessons in breathing from the diaphragm, rebirthing, some Yoga exercises, blowing balloons, blowing out candles, peak flow meters, coughing techniques, voice therapy, and many others encourage us to breathe more deeply. Some of these examples may seem to be innocuous occurrences in our daily life, but they set us on a dangerous course.

• Doctors, in the main, are not yet aware that breathing, like other physiological functions, has a normal functioning state, so they rarely check or treat it. They should examine this aspect of their patients every bit as carefully as they check pulse or blood pressure, temperature, or cholesterol level.

Every one of these points suggests that our knowledge of breathing, respiration, and its link to illness remains dangerously insufficient. It's clear that unless something dramatic is done to change the way we think, and the way we breathe, hyperventilation will remain a killer for the next generations. And, the many diseases and health conditions caused or exacerbated by hyperventilation will continue to plague the population.

But it's not all gloom and doom. For those of us who have already experienced or witnessed the extraordinary effects of Breath Connection, there is help at hand. We may be a small minority of the population at present, but word is spreading, and this program is set to change the way we view illness forever.

There are, already, hundreds of people whose lives have been radically and triumphantly changed by the growing new awareness of the dangers of hyperventilation. This is John's story:

JOHN

People tend to associate ME (myalgic encephalomyelitis) or chronic fatigue syndrome with women, but men can be vulnerable, too. John, a university student, enjoyed various sports in his leisure time and was reasonably fit. He drank socially and didn't smoke, but he had a tendency to regular colds and flu, and he took medicines for this, occasionally using a nasal spray at night.

After one particularly nasty bout of flu, he remained weak, giddy, and generally unwell for weeks. His doctor prescribed antibiotics and vitamin supplements but after further weeks of illness, further drugs, and further assurances from his GP that all would be well soon, he despaired. After months of the same debilitating symptoms, he was finally diagnosed as suffering from ME. By that time he was sleeping for up to 14 hours a day, had dropped out of his course, lost contact with most of his friends, and spent most of his few waking hours in bed. He had no strength to leave his bedroom, let alone even consider resuming his old lifestyle. John also found it difficult to read or concentrate and became both so angry with his doctor and depressed at life in general that he seriously considered suicide.

He soon began to have difficulty breathing—and it was this final symptom that saved him. John's mother saw an advertisement for a Breath Connection workshop and somehow John found the energy and motivation to attend. The first time he attended his Control Pause (CP) was a frightening 8 seconds. He was weak and pale after six months indoors, and his symptoms were as crippling as ever. Yet, after the second day, he began sleeping for only eight or nine hours a night and his muscular pains lessened. After a week, with his CP improving all the time, he began to go out walking and shopping. Less than two months later, John had resumed his studies and three months later was back playing basketball, his CP a very sound 45.

We'll be giving you lots of inspiring examples like John's story throughout our book, and they may just be the impetus you need to make changes that will affect the rest of your life.

Points to Remember

• Most people are inhaling more air than their bodies need. This has an adverse affect on the delicate balance between carbon dioxide and oxygen levels, triggering the compensatory defense mechanisms which we call *disease*. More than 200 disorders can be reversed or eased with correct breathing (the most common of which are listed in Appendix B).

• Your body needs a precise level of carbon dioxide for oxygen to reach its vital tissues and organs.

• Carbon dioxide was once considered to be a waste gas and a poison to the body. Professor Buteyko's discoveries herald a new appreciation of the important, indeed vital, role that it plays in health. The key to optimum well-being is the natural balance between oxygen and carbon dioxide.

• Much of the advice offered by medical experts, physiotherapists, sports trainers, and even some complementary therapists to breathe deeply has been based on scientific misunderstandings that have only been challenged relatively recently. Don't imagine the old rules are all still valid.

- Our CP (Control Pause) test can indicate if you are hyperventilating, whether or not you know it.
- The Breath Connection program exercises have been responsible for a 90 percent improvement in the condition of people with asthma and have contributed toward further dramatic improvement in the condition of people suffering from other illnesses.

3

Breath Connection Basics

Before we go on to discuss the exercises for individual health conditions, it is important that the basic Breath Connection techniques are clearly understood. The exercises that form the basis of the program are easy to understand and to implement, and within five days you will see outstanding benefits. The exercises can be adapted according to your individual needs, and with the help of a Breath Connection counselor, you can come up with the ideal formula for you. If you plan to practice the exercises from home, there are a few safety notes to consider. We'll discuss these alongside the basic exercises that form the treatment.

The most important part of the program is the Control Pause. It is both a test, a monitor, and a tool for controlling your breathing. Here's how it's done.

The Control Pause

Four to six liters of air per minute are all you need to supply your blood with oxygen. More than that, particularly if you are breathing deeply or erratically, can destabilize the central nervous, cardiovascular, immune, hormonal, excretory, and digestive systems. It can also lead to general fatigue and sleeping problems. It is very easy to breath more air per minute without seeming to be overbreathing, and most of us do it. As a result we are all, unknowingly, damaging our health on a regular basis.

To discover if you are unconsciously hyperventilating, try the Control Pause (CP) test. This simple exercise is central to the Breath Connection program.

1. Sit comfortably in an upright chair close to a clock with a second hand, or hold a stopwatch.
2. Relax and breathe in and out gently, mouth closed.
3. Pinch your nose with your fingers, after the exhalation.
4. Keeping your mouth closed, count how many seconds you can comfortably last before you need to inhale again.
5. Don't push yourself too hard. The accuracy of the test depends on you stopping before you reach the threshold of discomfort.
6. Remember: you are not holding your breath in, you are emptying your lungs and then counting.
7. When you breathe in again, try not to take in large gulps of air, control your breathing, keep your mouth closed.
8. Do *not* push your Control Pause above 60. This can only be done under the guidance of a Breath Connection Practitioner. These breathing exercises, like medication, must be administered correctly.

- A control pause of 50 to 60 seconds or more suggests that you are in excellent health. Holding for 25 seconds means that your health requires attention.
- If you can only manage 10 seconds or less, a serious

hyperventilation problem exists. This might already have manifested itself as asthma or some other illness.

• Anyone with a control pause of less than 30 seconds needs to follow the exercises outlined in this book. The exercises are necessary for your general health and well-being and will help to prevent the creation of a fertile environment for more than 200 different health disorders (see page 253 for a list of the most common ones).

Take 60 as the ideal Control Pause. Now divide that number by your own CP. The answer tells you how many people you are breathing for—or, more importantly, how severely you are threatening your health. If your CP is 20, divide that number into 60. The answer is 3, which means that you are, effectively, breathing 3 times as often as you should be, or breathing for 3 people.

If you have ever suffered from any sort of respiratory disorder, you may feel daunted at the prospect of modifying the way you breathe—tampering with something that seems absolutely natural. We promise you that it isn't difficult and it certainly isn't dangerous. In many societies, past and present, breathing is naturally shallow normally, that is, shallow in terms of how much air is taken in. People in such societies have never been taught to breathe deeply, and so did not develop bad breathing habits such as breathing through the mouth. Everyone breathes in a much healthier way. We should not assume that our norm is what is right for us, particularly in light of the fact that we are, in the West, decidedly less healthy than our Eastern neighbors.

Try to see correct breathing as a form of nutrition. Just imagine how much harm you would be doing to yourself if you were eating for two, three, four, or more people.

You must always interrupt your CP test if you feel at all uncomfortable. Shallow breathe for a few minutes and start again without pushing yourself. Never forget that our exercises are as powerful and effective as some conventional medicines, so please follow the instructions carefully and never push yourself to get a higher Control Pause.

Shallow Breathing

Shallow breathing is the opposite of deep breathing. It involves taking in small quantities of air. The best way to achieve shallow breathing is to be aware of your breathing and to consciously regulate the flow in and out of the nose. Nasal breathing is the key to correct breathing. When we breathe through our mouths, we take in too much oxygen and breathe out too much carbon dioxide, which upsets the balance of these essential gases in our bodies.

It has been established that people with breathing disorders, such as asthma, often have nasal problems, too, such as sinusitis, rhinitis, or polyps. Most nasal problems—such as asthma—are one of the body's defense mechanisms against overbreathing. Breath Connection can teach you to get rid of nasal problems, and you will also learn how to get rid of asthma, which is another facet of the same problem.

After two or three days of practicing Breath Connection, your nasal passages will open up—and stay open—if you continue to breathe correctly.

Unblocking Your Nose

It may seem impossible to consider shallow breathing, or breathing through your nose, if you have chronically blocked nasal passages. We have a quick-fix method for unblocking your nose, which will provide relief for a few minutes, or even hours. Once you have practiced Breath Connection for a couple of days, your nose will stay clear, and this exercise will be unnecessary. This is what you do:

- Breathe in and out normally.
- Pinch your nose with two fingers after the exhalation.
- When you can no longer comfortably hold your breath out, let go of your nose, but keep your mouth closed and carry on breathing through your nose, which will now be open.

Try to move around while pinching your nose—the added movement will increase the carbon dioxide levels in your blood even further, and we know that carbon dioxide is a natural bronchodilator.

Taping

It can be difficult to remember to breathe through your nose, which is why we recommend taping. It's not as draconian as it sounds! We recommend a special type of tape, 3M micropore mouth tape, which is available from pharmacists and hardware shops. This tape can be applied and removed easily and painlessly, and because it has tiny pores, or holes, you will not feel completely suffocated. We suggest that you tape your mouth with a small piece of tape, placed vertically over the lips, while you learn the techniques and throughout the program. Obviously, this may not be appropriate if you are in an office or out and about throughout the day, but it should certainly be undertaken while you are at home, whenever you are alone, and definitely while sleeping. Children in particular need to be reminded to breathe through their noses, and this is an easy way to set a good habit in place. If your child or children are resistant, perhaps all members of the family can take part, so he or she will feel more involved. Taping is not essential, but it definitely improves your progress.

Sleeping Techniques

Asthma becomes worse at night and in the early hours of the morning because the horizontal position of your body during sleep increases hyperventilation. Professor Buteyko believes that this is because the natural position of our bodies is upright. Lying flat on our backs is not the optimum position for our breathing to function normally.

When we sleep, our breathing starts out being low and shallow. However, as we slip into deeper sleep, our breathing becomes deeper and deeper. When we are lying down, our breathing increases, so that our levels of carbon dioxide go down. So, how should we sleep?

The more upright you are, the better. Sitting up is the ideal position, but we accept that it isn't very comfortable— or practical. However, if your asthma symptoms are very bad, you might want to consider it. The next best option is to position yourself on a high pile of pillows, which should rest under your head and shoulders.

Always sleep on your left side, with your legs pulled up to your chest. This fetal position has been proved to be the most effective position for sleeping, although the reason is unclear. If you find it uncomfortable, switch to your right-hand side, which is, ultimately, much better than sleeping on your back. Lying on your back and breathing through your mouth is the worst possible way you can sleep. According to Professor Buteyko, children should sleep on their tummies.

Professor Buteyko recommends sleeping on a hard bed, such as a futon, or one with a thin mattress, and suggests that we should aim to reduce our time sleeping by as much as possible. The less you can sleep, the better. Here are some other tips for getting a good night's sleep:

- Don't go to bed until you are so tired that you cannot do anything else but sleep.
- Don't go to bed just because it is bedtime. Wait until you are genuinely tired before retiring for the night.
- Don't go to bed during the day. If you have had a sleepless night, take a 20- to 30-minute nap, sitting in a chair.
- Make sure your mouth is closed while you sleep and tape your lips to ensure that it stays this way. Breathing through your nose at night can reduce phlegm, prevent snoring, and provide a much more refreshing sleep. Most importantly, however, it can prevent asthma attacks.

Professor Buteyko noted that Native American women used their fingers to ensure that the mouths of their children were closed when they slept, until the children developed the habit of breathing through their noses. Doctors of the time noted that these children were often healthier than their Colonial contemporaries.

Taking Your Pulse

Before and after Breath Connection exercises you will take your pulse. Your pulse is a sure measure of the state of your health, and it's important that you learn how to measure it. Sit quietly for a few seconds before following these steps.

A pulse means that blood is circulating in the body. Check for a pulse:

- On the thumb side of the wrist, about 1.5 cm above the wrist crease and about 1.5 cm in from the side of the wrist.
- At the carotid artery in the neck, which runs up either side of the back of the Adam's apple. You'll find the

Taking your pulse

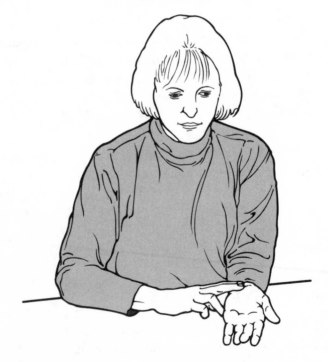

pulse in the hollow between the Adam's apple and the neck muscle.

1. Check for a pulse by pressing two fingers on either of the pulse points (not both). Never use your thumb to take a pulse since it has a pulse of its own.
2. If you do not feel something immediately, press a little deeper and move your fingers around gently to find the pulse point.

In general, 70 beats per minute indicates that your health is good. Up to 80 it is probably fair, but 100 is too high. There are very few people whose health is fine, even if they have a high pulse rate and body temperature, but don't take the risk that you may be one of them. When you normalize your breathing, your whole system becomes more efficient and less stressed—and so normalizes the heartbeat. Checking your pulse rate before and after doing the Control Pause exercises will demonstrate how breathing correctly has a direct bearing on circulation. As your CP goes up, your pulse rate will come down. You will be checking your pulse regularly to ensure that this happens. It is a very good way to gauge the effect of the exercises.

The Exercises

The Breath Connection program is made up of a series of exercises in which you learn to control your breathing. The exercises are suggested according to the severity of your symptoms, the condition from which you might be suffering, and what you hope to achieve from the program. In general, the exercises involve the Control Pause, which is used both to monitor your condition and to help control your breathing, shallow breathing techniques, and, at various stages, taking your pulse.

The program also involves learning to breathe through your nose and making adjustments to your day-to-day breathing techniques in order to learn normal breathing. In Breath Connection, you are taught to breathe less air, which is considered to be normal breathing. Abnormal breathing is the cause of many diseases; normal breathing, the Breath Connection way, will both improve your health and well-being. You'll start to see changes after only a few days. Now, let's begin.

4

Breath Connection for Adults with Asthma

Every asthmatic is an individual and no one series of steps will work for everyone. In this chapter, we look at the special needs of adult asthmatics and emphysemics, whether your levels of distress are high or relatively low. Later on, we look at the different problems that children and their caregivers face and the separate needs of those whose lives are blighted by related disorders.

Here, we address the appalling symptoms experienced during an asthma attack. Sufferers will be more than familiar with that terrifyingly severe shortness of breath, the pain, the panic, and the fear that you are going to die. An asthma attack can also be frightening to witness, but unless you are a sufferer there can be little understanding of the severity of the problem, and the overwhelming dread and fear that it produces.

When a person is breathing normally, the bronchotubes are open and there is no asthma. If we begin to overbreathe/hyperventilate and start exhaling too much carbon dioxide, the bronchotubes narrow in order to prevent the body from losing so much carbon dioxide. In an asthma attack, a bronchospasm occurs, and the hyperventilation can become even more pronounced. After using a reliever, the bronchotubes

A vicious cycle in asthma

1

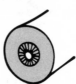

Normal breathing
Bronchotubes are open—no asthma

2

Asthmatic's breathing
Bronchotubes are narrowed (hyperventilation)

3

During asthma attack
Bronchospasm—hyperventilation is even greater

4

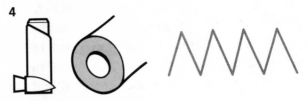

After use of reliever
Bronchotubes are open but hyperventilation is even worse

5

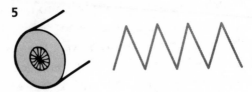

New bronchospasm and the need to use reliever again

are opened, the asthma symptoms are relieved, but the underlying problem of hyperventilation is even worse. A new bronchospasm forms and the asthmatic needs to use the reliever again. The vicious cycle is complete.

But, this cycle can be broken, and in a few short days you can experience huge relief. In this chapter, we provide invaluable advice on self-care for adult asthmatics. If you don't suffer from a respiratory illness, turn to Chapter 9, where we provide tips on Breath Connection for general health.

We begin with a word about the drugs and medication that you may well have relied upon for some time. Understanding them and correct usage is essential to your recovery.

Drugs and Medication

Some drugs, judiciously used, are helpful. Taken in partnership with the Breath Connection program, some medication can ease your symptoms as you travel the road to recovery. But remember: Any drug has the strength and power to damage as well as heal. Now is the time to assess your actual needs and decide whether a prescription that may have been appropriate for you years ago is relevant to your present condition. Every illness progresses, and there is every likelihood that the drugs you are taking now are unnecessary or even inappropriate. Perhaps you do need to continue with the same type of medication, but you should certainly query whether the dosage is right for your present needs. Consider whether these drugs have actually made you feel better over the years, or have they merely staved off attacks?

When you break a leg or arm you need to be protected by a plaster cast for a short period. You don't need that shield for the rest of your life. Try to think of prescribed asthma drugs in the same way.

Read this section on medication for asthma, emphysema, and other respiratory conditions with care. Be optimistic and try not to depend on crutches that you may no longer need. Pick up a crutch, by all means, when you are very weary, but learn not to depend on it as an everyday prop. You will see how a dependency can actually encourage the development, rather than elimination, of other disorders.

We know that some drugs and medicines, correctly administered, can be vital. But the sad fact is that sometimes drugs can actually aggravate asthma. We see conventional asthma medication as a very useful stop-gap, on which you can rely in times of need, while you learn the basics of the Breath Connection program and come to appreciate its fuller and longer-term benefits. Little by little, as your symptoms of asthma decrease, you can reduce your drug intake. It goes without saying that no medication should be discontinued or reduced without consulting your doctor, but we are confident that the Breath Connection program will make such a dramatic change that even your doctor will have to agree that drugs may no longer be necessary.

Many doctors may not have been aware of the Breath Connection program, and it is up to us to ensure that they are educated about this revolutionary system. While you are learning the techniques, your doctor can alter your drug intake as he or she sees fit. In partnership with Breath Connection techniques, some carefully prescribed drugs can be very helpful. Explain to your doctor what you are doing, and let him or her witness the results. You will find that your need for medication is reduced or even entirely nonexistent once you have started the program. Your body will be more balanced and in control, and the need for external treatment may well be completely unnecessary.

Understanding Your Drugs

All drugs have side effects. If you take an aspirin for your headache, the chances are that one or more of your other senses will be dulled. It's easy to ignore niggling side effects when you have been taking an asthma-related medicine for years. Indeed, the medicine may well have become a placebo. You may need to use a little amateur psychology to analyze this: Do you take those medicines because you know they will help you or because you subconsciously believe that they are a kind of insurance against an attack?

In the future, think more carefully about why and when you take that medication. Remember that taking drugs automatically could lead to further problems with hyperventilation and, in turn, lead to a stay in the hospital where further drugs will probably be administered. This is the cycle that we aim to break.

Most drugs are prescribed at the same dosage each day, occasionally at specified times. We do not agree with this method of treatment. We believe that as a patient's health or symptoms improve, the drug intake should be reduced. At the very least it should be varied, depending upon how you feel from day to day. A single prescribed level should be maintained only if you cannot see any change in your condition over a long period of time. Even then, don't let that situation carry on indefinitely. If you are chronically ill, and your medication has not made any improvement, chances are that the drug is not doing anything at all. Remember that all pharmaceutical drugs, including adrenaline, are prescribed to ease symptoms. They are not created to address the causes of illness, only its physical manifestations. The causes of many chronic illnesses remain unknown, despite the fact that the majority of them are treated regularly with prescription drugs.

Adrenaline, in particular, is used regularly for the treatment of asthma. Adrenaline derives from the adrenal cortex, a gland that produces natural corticosteroids. Asthmatics cannot produce enough of this natural steroid and often rely on synthetic substitutes. Experiments in Australia show that patients who follow Breath Connection are able to reduce their intake of artificial steroids by half. This clearly indicates that our bodies can learn to produce sufficient levels of this natural steroid on their own. Professor Buteyko maintains that the need for synthetic steroids is a direct result of hyperventilation, and the fact that the body produces its own, once it is back in balance, supports this view.

Shocking as it might seem, steady use of bronchodilators could worsen your asthma in the long run and could even be fatal. Recent asthma epidemics in the relatively clean environments of Australia and New Zealand have been attributed to the overuse of nebulizers.

KEY TERMS

• *Bronchodilators* are drugs prescribed to widen the bronchioles and improve breathing. There are three main groups of bronchodilators: sympathomimetics, anticholinergics, and xanthine drugs, which are related to caffeine. Corticosteroids are also used to reduce inflammation and suppress allergic reactions.

• Bronchodilators can either be taken when they are needed in order to relieve an attack of breathlessness that is in progress, or on a regular basis to prevent such attacks from occurring.

• Sympathomimetic drugs are mainly used for the rapid relief of breathlessness; anticholinergic drugs and xanthine drugs are used in the long term.

• Bronchodilator drugs act by relaxing the muscles surrounding the bronchioles.

• Sympathomimetic and anticholinergic drugs achieve this by interfering with the nerve signals passed to the muscles through the autonomic nervous system. Xanthine drugs are believed to relax the muscle in the bronchioles by their direct effect on the muscle fibers, although their precise action is unknown.

• Bronchodilator drugs usually improve breathing within a few minutes of administration.

• Corticosteroids usually start to increase the sufferer's capacity for exercise within a few days.

• All of these drugs have side effects: Sympathomimetic drugs stimulate a branch of the autonomic nervous system that controls heart rate and they may sometimes cause palpitations and trembling; anticholinergic drugs cause a dry mouth, blurred vision, and difficulty in passing urine; xanthine drugs may cause headaches and nausea. Corticosteroids may cause water retention, swelling, and an increase in blood pressure. They reduce the effect of insulin and may cause problems in diabetics, even producing the disease in susceptible individuals. They suppress the immune system, increasing the susceptibility to infection, and suppress symptoms of infectious disease. With long-term use, they can cause muscle wasting, peptic ulcers, osteoporosis, easy bruising, and a fat pad on the back.

• Inhalers or "puffers" release a small dose of a bronchodilator drug when pressed.

• Insufflation cartridges deliver larger amounts of the drug than inhalers and are easier to use because the drug is taken in as you breathe normally.

• Nebulizers pump compressed air through a solution of drug to produce a fine mist which is inhaled through a face mask. They deliver large doses of the drug to the lungs, rapidly relieving breathing difficulty.

• Ventilators are machines used to stimulate breathing in hospital.

COMMON DRUGS

Sympathomimetics

Bambuterol

Eformoterol

Ephedrine

Epinephrine

Fenoterol

Isoprenaline

Pirbuterol

Reproterol

Rimiterol

Salbutamol

Salmeterol

Terbutaline

Tulobuterol

Anticholinergics

Atropine

Ipratropium bromide

Oxitropium

Xanthines
   Theophylline/aminophylline

Corticosteroids
   Beclomethasone
   Budesonide
   Fluticasone
   Prednisolone

Other Drugs
   Antihistamines
   Ketotifen
   Nedocromil
   Sodium cromoglycate

There are some startling statistics, which bear out our worries:

- In 1930, when adrenaline first appeared, there was an increase in asthma-related deaths.
- Mortality was further increased following the widespread prescription and use of Isoprenaline, a bronchodilator, in 1960.
- Sudden respiratory arrests were reported among young asthmatics who had taken Salmetorol (Serevent) and in 1996 a group of Canadian scientists found that even as few as two puffs a day from a bronchodilator—about 200 milligrams—not only worsened the condition of asthma patients but contributed to a higher incidence of cataracts and glaucoma problems in asthmatics.

- According to a 1989 study, asthma mortality increased to epidemic proportions in New Zealand and was linked to inhaled Fenoterol.
- A 1990 study claimed that inhaled steroids were contributing to many psychiatric and endocrine disorders.

We offer these facts not to alarm you, but to point out the very real dangers of some drugs. It may help you to decide that the Breath Connection program, which uses only natural means by which to treat asthma and related conditions, is a healthier and safer alternative to long-term drug use. One of the aims of our treatment is to help you to reduce any existing drug dependency, and in consultation with your doctor you could soon be able to set aside your bronchodilator and steroid intake.

In our overstretched health service, GPs (general practitioners) are usually very busy. If your doctor does not have the time to discuss things as fully as you would like, we offer the following facts for you to consider for yourself. With this knowledge, you can consult your doctor about making possible changes.

Bronchodilators

These contain natural substances as well as manufactured drugs and have an honorable history going back to a Chinese doctor, Ma Huang, who devised one using the herb *Ephedra*, more than 4,000 years ago. Hippocrates, the father of modern medicine, was the first physician to identify asthma in the West. He called it *asthma*, which in translation means "hard to breathe." The first modern-day bronchodilators, which included ephedrine and adrenaline, were devised about 70 years ago. Before that, whisky, caffeine, tobacco, and chloroform had all been used to treat paroxysms of the bronchial tubes. Let us hope that the Breath Connection will in time be seen as another—but better—example of science's fragmented leaps and bounds.

Steroids

The steroids used for asthma and similar conditions are called *corticosteroids* and should not be confused with anabolic steroids, which are sometimes illegally taken by athletes to improve performance. When a medical pioneer was awarded the Nobel Prize for medicine for his discovery of steroid-related drugs and their anti-inflammatory effects, there was a rush to embrace them. People who had suffered for years from arthritis, skin disorders, chronic pain, and indeed asthma did not stop to query their possible side effects and the long-term damage they can produce. Diabetes sufferers gained relief and there was an almost universal, if hasty, welcome for the drugs and their spin-offs, many of which were lifesaving. Then came the backlash. Artificial steroids given to asthmatics and others produced some horrific side effects, including puffy faces, excess weight, excess facial hair for women, ulcers, osteoporosis, and serious problems for diabetics, including blindness, deafness, and memory loss. The regular prescription of most forms of steroid was halted for some time, while the medical profession reconsidered their uses. Over this period, nasal sprays and some skin creams were still widely available.

The overuse of artificial steroids suppresses the body's ability to produce natural steroids. Some people, particularly asthmatics, develop such a severe steroid dependency that they need to resort to drugs as their needs exceed their body's ability to produce the natural versions. The increased dosages and increasing use of these drugs will, over time, harm sufferers far more than they will help them. Some doctors have been unable to see the difference between the natural and unnatural steroids and have unwittingly colluded in the dangerous dependency of their patients. When the glands cease to produce natural steroids, due to artificial interference, the adrenal cortex is affected.

Other doctors, who may have been warned of the dangers of overprescribing steroids, actually underprescribe, which also puts their patients in danger. Steroids can be an effective, short-term treatment for a variety of illnesses, but their use must be assessed on a regular basis and regulated constantly.

Furthermore, few doctors actually understand how steroids work. Typically, oral steroids are prescribed for use in the morning, on the basis that they will tune in to the rhythms of the body. However, most asthmatic patients are at most risk early in the day, and since these types of steroids normally kick in after about six hours, they are virtually useless. Steroids are meant to be used on a preventative basis and not used to relieve an attack. It would be far better if they were taken at night so that problems early the next day can be avoided.

And why do doctors so often reduce the dosage of steroids by one tablet every three days, as if this treatment were set in stone? Why not every day, every two days, or every seven days? Surely these adjustments should be made after observing a patient's individual needs, which can change daily. The diagram below may help to explain things.

Steroid medication

a) Graphically, the steroid policy for a typical patient looks like this:

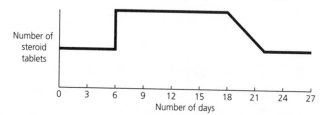

A doctor will increase the dose to 6–8 tablets in a day. The patient is then maintained on this high dosage for 10–12 days, after which it is gradually reduced by 1 tablet every 3 days, bringing it down to nothing. Professor Buteyko believes steroid intake should be adjusted for the particular condition of the patient in a more flexible way. In a typical case, with this sudden increase and decrease in dosage, the patient's health will improve and deteriorate just as quickly.

b) Often asthmatic patients have to go to the hospital where they can be given 200–1,000 mg of steroids. Graphically, this looks like this:

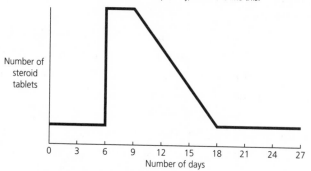

The patient is given a very high dose suddenly. When he or she leaves the hospital, the dose is reduced to nothing, endangering the patient's condition.

A Steroid Case

Let's take the case of an imaginary patient who visits his doctor and is prescribed oral steroids. Until now, the patient has been taking four puffs from an inhaler on most days. This amounts to a total daily dosage of one milligram of steroids (even more if the steroid prescribed was Beclomethasone).

He is now advised to take six to eight tablets, amounting to 30 or 40 milligrams daily, and typically advised to decrease this intake by one tablet every three days. This would likely produce the following scenario:

- The patient has now been prescribed 30 or 40 times more steroids than he has been used to (and even more if the choice of drug was Beclomethasone).
- The patient reduces this dosage by one tablet, or five milligrams, every three days. Therefore, he will take eight tablets on days one to three, seven on days four to six, and six tablets on days seven to nine, and so on over 21 days until he is taking no tablets at all.

Over three weeks, the patient has taken 128 tablets of oral steroids, each containing five milligrams. This means that he has ingested a total of 640 milligrams, a huge amount compared to the 21 milligrams he would have been taking over the previous three weeks.

In the first three days, the patient's body must adapt to an increase of 117 milligrams of steroids. This is cause for concern and raises the following questions: On what basis did the doctor prescribe the original four puffs a day? Why does this prescription tend to be offered fairly universally? If you suffer from diabetes your doctor will measure your blood sugar level and prescribe correct dosages of insulin accordingly. Patients' needs should be met on an individual basis. This practice has rarely, if ever, been considered for asthmatics.

Why was the new dosage of steroids increased 40-fold to cope with the problem? If a diabetic's blood sugar level suddenly jumped, his doctor would be unlikely to increase his insulin intake so dramatically.

It is easy to overdose on steroids, and their side effects are evident on even lower dosages, taken over a longer period of time. Administered correctly, there is no doubt that steroids can save lives. However, Professor Buteyko believes that the frequent and improper use of steroids is the cause of great discomfort and has even contributed to death. Not surprisingly, many people are becoming worried about taking them at all. His policy on steroids is very clear:

• Correctly prescribed steroids are a very effective means of preventing asthma attacks, subsequent deterioration, and even death from asthma.

• Ignorance in understanding their importance, reluctance, or refusal to take steroids can be fatal, as can medical negligence in failing to prescribe the right dosage.

• The vast majority of doctors do not know how steroids work; how to select correct dosages; how to modify dosage on a daily basis; or how or when to increase, decrease, or maintain levels of steroid consumption when a patient's condition worsens. Neither do they know how to normalize natural steroid production, overcome the resulting steroid deficiency, and get the patient off artificial steroids permanently.

Professor Buteyko's discovery includes a thorough understanding of drugs and can help you to both stay alive and enjoy a greater level of freedom in your everyday life.

We can show you how not only the dosage but the side effects of steroids can be minimized once your individual and precise needs have been gauged, and we can show you how you can soon stop taking them altogether. These drugs play a very similar role in the life of an asthmatic as insulin does in the life of a diabetic. When the body hyperventilates, it stops producing natural steroids, so manufactured ones are required. But once you have learned not to overbreathe and your own natural steroids are being produced, prescribed medicine becomes redundant. With our help and that of your doctor, this is achievable. During this interim period it is essential to follow Professor Buteyko's principles and to carry on taking your steroids, but only under careful guidance.

The Peak Flow Meter

A peak flow meter is a device used to measure the volume of your forced expiration. The idea is that you blow into it as hard as you can to produce a reading that tells you your ability to blow out air. The higher the reading, the greater the volume of air and the better the result, according to doctors.

This device is familiar to every asthmatic and emphysema sufferer and in our view it is a thoroughly worthless piece of equipment: misleading, harmful, and only good for showing how strongly you can exhale. Even then it gives out imprecise measurements and can, in fact, induce asthmatic symptoms. Few doctors query the usefulness of peak flow meters and they can't explain why they can sometimes trigger an asthma-like effect. Attempts made by doctors and patients alike to maintain good peak flow figures are doomed to fail because trying to increase peak flow figures artificially leads, in every case, to hyperventilation. As we know, hyperventilation leads to asthma, the need for drugs, and a destructive cycle.

When you blow into the device, you blow out a great deal of carbon dioxide, which tells your body to defend itself by constricting the bronchotubes. This is the reason why asthmatics and others with breathing disorders experience wheezing, discomfort, coughing, and tightness of the chest after blowing out air. It is pointless to try to improve your peak flow figures without understanding the reasons for your problem. We know that asthma is caused by hyperventilation, which causes inadequate carbon dioxide to reach the body. A peak flow meter can cause hyperventilation.

Reconditioning and normalizing breathing patterns should be the first goal of every asthmatic—and a peak flow meter does nothing to effect this. We suggest you throw away your peak flow meter—now.

Watchpoints

Asthmatics should take special care to avoid attack in the following situations, particularly before they have reconditioned their breathing by following our program:

- When leaving a warm room for a cold street, or vice versa.
- When showering. Rapid changes in water temperature have been known to trigger attacks.
- Talking for long periods, which can encourage you to take in more air than you need. Schoolteachers, telephone salespeople, and anyone who needs to speak frequently as they work should be especially careful. See page 222 for techniques on breathing correctly when you talk.
- Dusting and making beds. Dust and mites, which can encourage attacks in asthmatics, thrive in even the most carefully laundered duvets and mattresses. Try and get someone else to make the bed or be sure to keep your mouth closed when you do so. Think about buying a special mattress cover or investing in one of the more powerful vacuum cleaners.

• Watch your diet. Asthmatic problems often become worse in cold weather, particularly if you have had colds or flu. Make sure you are getting lots of vitamin C and zinc, which can encourage the health of the immune system, and take the herb Echinacea, which has been proved both to boost immunity and reduce the duration of viral symptoms.

• Take care when you are flying. A pressurized cabin can play havoc with breathing. Concentrate on your breath control for several days before you fly and especially on the day of travel, right up to boarding the plane.

Remember:

• In all situations that can trigger an asthma attack, you must control your breathing. If you experience any asthma symptoms or find yourself hyperventilating, stay calm and concentrate on the breathing exercises.

• Sleep as upright as possible, supporting yourself with several firm pillows. There is always a danger that the pillows might move during a restless night, but begin by propping yourself in the right position, and settled on the left side of the body (see pages 52–53).

• Concentrate on your Breath Connection exercises before you go to bed, particularly if you have had a stressful day or have been in situations that normally trigger an attack. If your breathing is under control, you are much less likely to be wakened by an attack or to suffer one in the morning.

Special Note
Before embarking on the Breath Connection program in this book you should ascertain whether you are suffering from

any of the illnesses and disorders noted in Appendix B (see page 253). Some conditions are too complicated to be addressed without the guidance of a qualified practitioner or specialist. In the Resources section, we tell you how to find a reputable practitioner in your area. Always remember that the Breath Connection techniques, although simple, are very powerful and should only be practiced carefully. Never deviate from the guidelines supplied here and if you are in doubt, or feel uncomfortable at any point, take expert advice.

5

Breath Connection for Mild Asthma

Mild asthma can be as disrupting and distressing as more serious asthma, although it may not hold the same risks for the sufferer. Everything is relative, of course, and it is very likely that while you are in the grip of an attack, your symptoms may seem anything but mild, even if you have been diagnosed with a mild condition. Everyone has a different ability to cope with illness, just as everyone has different pain thresholds. Chances are, whether your asthma is mild or severe, you are suffering a great deal and are unlikely to be relieved or comforted by the fact that your condition is *mild*. We are aware that all asthma causes suffering and can lead to more serious illness. Breath Connection can ease that suffering.

We promise that within a few days you will be less dependent upon medication, and that your breathlessness and wheezing will be reduced if you follow the program for a week. Perhaps the most important result of the program is the fact that you will be able to control your asthma, rather than your asthma controlling you. As your body and your emotional health become stronger, you will begin to feel more in control of your life, and your health and well-being can be improved immeasurably.

We call your asthma mild if you

- Have never had any critical, life-threatening attacks
- Have never been hospitalized for asthma
- Have never used oral steroids, such as Prednisone
- Do not use Severent or a nebulizer
- Experience symptoms less than three or four times a day
- Can gain relief from a single puff of an inhaler

If one or more of these points does not apply to you, we would consider your asthma to be severe.

The importance of the balance between oxygen and carbon dioxide has been made clear. Carbon dioxide beneficially affects almost every organ and system in the body and can help to stop asthma from gaining any ground. If they could, pharmaceutical companies would undoubtedly bottle carbon dioxide, and there would be a large-scale fight for the patent. But carbon dioxide is free, and in order to experience its unique benefits, you need only learn a series of breathing exercises that will allow you to access it. Do your Control Pauses (see page 48) and breathe shallowly, with your mouth closed, to prevent this priceless gas from escaping. You will see results within days.

Another great benefit of the Breath Connection program—which is useful for all asthmatics and emphysemics, as well as everyone concerned about the general state of their health—is that it acts as an invaluable monitor. Your Control Pauses will tell you a great deal about your general state of health and help you to chart your daily progress. This can be enormously comforting for sufferers of any condition. If you are on top of your health and can gauge the results of the program, you will feel in control. You will never again have to fear illness in the same way. You will never again have to ask yourself "Am I really well?" "Am I more vulnerable than others to a life-threatening illness?" "Can I look forward to a long and healthy retirement?"

The Control Pause exercises will let you know in advance when things are wrong and help you to take control before early problems take hold. You will be much more confident and able to deal with health worries effectively.

It's simple! When your CP goes up, it indicates that your health is improving. When it goes down, take note and seek advice before any problem becomes more severe.

Preparing for Breath Connection

Everyone who is mildly asthmatic should prepare for Breath Connection by doing the following:

- Using their inhaler only when they cannot breathe.
- Getting used to breathing through the nose only, even when engaged in sporting activity. If this is impossible, take a break from the sport until your asthma is under control.
- Concentrating on learning how to shallow breathe.
- Making a habit of sitting comfortably and learning to relax.
- Beginning to breathe in more and more shallowly until your breathing is very gentle and quiet.
- Taking heart when things become difficult. It is worth persevering. Poor breathing can be changed much more easily than most bad habits.

The Technique

Each morning before breakfast (do this even if you are not hungry enough to eat any), sit and relax for five minutes. You can accomplish a whole series of breathing exercises while listening to the radio or some music.

1. Check your pulse over one minute and then practice a Control Pause.
2. Start shallow breathing for five minutes, and then do another Control Pause exercise.
3. Take a further five minutes for shallow breathing out.
4. Then, breathe in, breathe out, and hold your breath for the length of your last Control Pause, plus five seconds.
5. Now breathe lightly for five minutes.

Technique for mild asthmatics

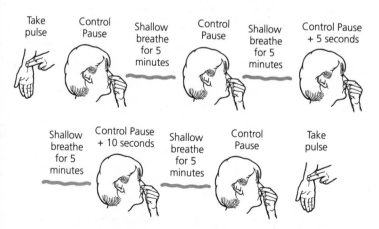

Practice this 3 times per day before meals until your symptoms disappear.

6. Breathe in, breathe out, and hold your breath out for the length of your last Control Pause, plus 10 seconds.
7. Finally, breathe shallowly for five minutes, then check your Control Pause and your pulse.

This type of breathing may have been a little faster than the type of breathing you are used to, but remember that the crucial thing is the reduced volume of air, not the speed at which you breathe. It is healthy and normal for you to feel slightly different to begin with, as your body adjusts to your new habit.

The whole morning exercise will take about 25 minutes, and we recommend that you try to repeat the sequence before lunch and your evening meal.

It's also a good idea to go through this cycle again, about an hour before you go to bed. Try to avoid eating anything for a couple of hours before each short session.

This series of exercises gives you a great start to the day and allows you to end each day feeling relaxed and calm. You can look forward to a peaceful, relaxing sleep.

Don't hesitate to do a course with a Breath Connection practitioner if you have any difficulty understanding these routines or putting them into practice. All counselors have been trained to understand, and be sympathetic toward, the problems of people who are unused to carving out spaces of time in their lives. They will offer encouragement and guidance to allow you to do so.

Key Points

- Get used to breathing less deeply than you are used to breathing.

- Keep your mouth closed, unless you are eating, speaking, or drinking.
- Close your mouth with special micropore tape (see page 51) before sleep or when you are alone at home.
- Keep up with your preventative medication. Don't stop or reduce steroids until your Breath Connection counselor has given you the OK, in consultation with your doctor.
- Practice your exercises regularly—this means three to four times a day for the next five days.
- Don't overeat or oversleep, and try to avoid sleeping on your back. Try to arrange things so that you are propped up to sleep on your left side.
- Refer to the dietary guidelines in Chapter 12, which will enhance your recovery.
- Don't eat a protein meal in the evening (see page 193).
- Don't push your Control Pause over 60.
- When you finish your Control Pause and breathe in again, keep your mouth closed and try not to take in large gulps of air. Control your breathing.

You will soon find that your asthma symptoms are reduced, and you will need to resort less frequently to your bronchodilator. Use the chart on page 243 to document your weekly progress. If or when asthma symptoms reappear, you can take immediate action to overcome the attack (see the following section).

Overcoming Asthma Attacks

Many people have some advance warning of an attack, and it is important that you go through a single set of steps before one can set in. Try the following:

1. Sit down.
2. Take your pulse and do the Control Pause.
3. Shallow breathe for four or five minutes.
4. Repeat the Control Pause.
5. Take your pulse again.

If you are able to overcome the attack with Breath Connection, shallow breathe for another 10 minutes. You will not need to reach for your puffer if your asthma attack has been relieved. However, if it hasn't, use your puffer and continue to breathe shallowly for 10 minutes. You can repeat these exercises as often as you need to, whenever you want to regulate your breathing or stave off an attack.

Diary of a Mild Asthmatic

The following diary gives you an example of what a mild asthmatic might expect during five days on the Breath Connection program. Responses will differ between individuals, and different people will benefit in different ways. Every person will also progress at their own pace, so don't be alarmed if your progress is unlike what we describe here.

Day One
The number of relievers necessary will be reduced, and you can expect to sleep better. You will find it easier to unblock your nose, and there will less breathlessness and fewer asthma symptoms.

Day Two
You will need even less relief from your regular medication. There will be less mucus in the nose. Appetite will have been

stimulated in people who are underweight, and overweight people will experience less hunger. Breathlessness and the ability to overcome symptoms quickly and efficiently will be improved.

Day Three

Your breath control will be noticeably better, and all of the previously mentioned areas will continue to improve. You will be particularly aware of the changes as you walk upstairs. Coughing may be suppressed. Your use of the puffer will have become occasional and your Control Pause will be stronger.

Day Four

There will be a further improvement in your Control Pause and in your overall condition. Your nose should remain unblocked all day. Your weight will begin to stabilize.

Day Five

By now, the overall improvement in, and control of, your asthma will be about 70 percent, with a similar reduction in the number of times you need to use your bronchodilators. You should also see a 70 percent improvement in your ability to prevent many of the symptoms of allergy, asthma, and sinusitis, among other things. Your mouth will remain closed naturally when you are not talking or eating.

In a few weeks' time, your improvement will be dramatic and your Control Pause will be much higher. Your immune system and nervous system will begin to function better and you should experience an increased sense of well-being. You will have more control over your emotions and, if you wish, you will be able to take part in nonaggressive sport without the need for drugs. Dependence upon bronchodilator drugs will have been greatly lessened over the weeks on the program. Necessary weight loss or weight gain will have become steady, and your sleep will be improved. Best of all, your sense of well-being will be enhanced and you will, perhaps for the first time in a long, long time, feel in control of your life.

6

Breath Connection for Severe Asthma

For those of you who suffer from severe asthma, one of the most difficult things to overcome is fear. Many of you have been rushed to the hospital in an emergency or have suffered a life-threatening attack, and it is undoubtedly hard to get over the overwhelming emotion that you associate with an asthma attack, and, indeed, your health in general. People who suffer from any known or unknown fear tend to cling to the known and avoid taking chances that could put them in any physical or emotional danger. We know, therefore, that it may be difficult for you to adapt to the program without some reservations. We ask you to trust us and allow us to take you through the exercises that can not only ease your suffering, but help you to shed your fear forever.

First of all, read the preceding chapter aimed at mild asthmatics, because much of the material written there will be helpful for you, too. Your case will differ from that of a mild asthmatic in that you will need to be ready for action at any time, and you may not have the same warning that an attack is imminent.

We do understand that severe asthmatics live in fear that the enemy might strike at any time—during a business meeting, while traveling, during a family celebration, especially if it involves a heavy meal, or even during a quiet period at home. Stress isn't always the trigger for the awful gasping spasms that can send you into the hospital. Extremes of weather may also be worrying for you. Even making a quick dash to answer the telephone, or running upstairs because you feel strong that day, can lead toward the kind of attack that all asthmatics dread.

If every simple little act of everyday life is loaded with potential risk, it is very hard to plan a normal existence. If fear dogs your every breath and step, your quality of life is seriously reduced. Even going into the hospital, itself a stressful experience, can exacerbate things. Many sufferers report that the concern of family and friends heightens their feelings of fear and helplessness, and you may feel that you have no control to change a situation that is continually spiralling in a downward direction. Your current medication may well give you both temporary relief and an illusion of control over things as you struggle to overcome serious attacks, but it is not curing your asthma. In reality, it is restricting your ability to make the most of your potential and to enjoy the full life you deserve.

We call your asthma severe if you answer yes to any of these questions:

- Have you experienced respiratory arrest, clinical death, lung collapse, or a life-threatening asthma attack that you were unable to treat on your own with the drugs that you had on hand?
- Do you have to use nebulizers, Serevent, or take more than three puffs from an inhaler every day?
- Do you need to use oral steroids every day or in a series of courses?
- Is your Control Pause less than 10 seconds?

- Apart from your asthma, do you suffer from any of the following: diabetes, a heart or kidney condition, epilepsy, high blood pressure, hypoglycemia, or emphysema?

A single affirmative answer means that you have what we classify as being *severe* asthma. If you have said yes to more than one, you will have even more to gain from practicing the Breath Connection methods.

JOANNE AND JENNY

Joanne and Jenny, 15-year-old twins, came to us about nine years ago. They had been asthmatic since birth and their condition was then regarded as being severe. They had been robbed of many of the pleasures of childhood and now they were being deprived of most of the freedoms of youth. Unable to attend normal school, they were taught at home. Even a few steps to the family car for an outing sometimes took an agonizing 20 minutes and they had been hospitalized at least 50 times in their short lives.

When they first started at a Breath Connection workshop, the girls couldn't manage the walking exercises that most five-year-olds accomplish very easily, but they had the will to progress and within four or five days they were spurring each other on with the tempting idea that they could soon be attending parties, instead of being trapped at home. Two months later their father, a ship's doctor, returned from a long voyage and found the twins playing volleyball in the back garden. He was astonished but naturally delighted to see how far and how fast they had progressed since he had seen them last.

You really can breathe your way out of this prison of devastating illness. It will take some effort and time but, as many who have already taken part in our program will testify, it is well worth it. Right from the start you will experience an improved sense of well-being that will encourage you to persevere. As your confidence grows, so will your control—until you are the master of this condition. Your need for medication will reduce steadily until the point that you find yourself being categorized as *mildly* asthmatic. As your breathing becomes more balanced your body will no longer depend upon asthma as a defense mechanism against its loss of carbon dioxide. For the first time in your life, perhaps, you will feel free. Progress for some patients is astonishingly fast. Others need a little more time. Don't lose heart—everyone gets there in the end.

The chart on pages 244–245 should be completed regularly and, as the days go by, it will be all the proof you need that your recovery is under way. You will see that by changing your breathing patterns you have the power to influence the severity of your asthma and the tools with which to cure it.

TONY

A successful and dynamic businessman, Tony did not want to admit that the asthma he had suffered since childhood was severe. He considered it mild, even though he was taking up to 20 puffs of Ventolin on bad days. He had been prescribed steroids but didn't bother to take them as he felt they offered no relief and he was, in any case, worried about side effects. He accepted that two puffs of Serevent in the morning and another at night could be helpful but realized that it was only giving symptomatic relief and not getting to the root cause of his asthma. He doubted if any treatment could do that.

Tony's diet was quite sensible: He drank only in moderation, exercised regularly, and didn't smoke. He had once had a severe asthma attack during a business trip abroad, and he dreaded a recurrence, knowing that changes in climate and extra stress could exacerbate things.

During one long flight, a head cold passed to his throat and bronchi and this time countless puffs of Ventolin brought no relief. A heavy restaurant dinner was followed by several frightening hours during which he fought for breath and Tony eventually called an ambulance to his hotel. He made a good recovery after receiving oxygen, nebulizers, IV aminophylline, and steroids but was advised to remain in the hospital under supervision, taking oral steroids because his oxygen level was so low. It was this experience that convinced Tony that his asthma wasn't so mild after all and led him to Breath Connection when he returned to Britain.

He embarked on the program with commitment and enthusiasm and after only three days was using just two puffs of Ventolin and none of his prescribed Serevent. He was advised to get out of the habit of puffing Ventolin automatically before sport, sex, walking upstairs, stressful meetings, or going to bed. He soon learned that he could do everything he normally did without hyperventilating or needing Ventolin. He also learned how to control his asthma by subtly adjusting all aspects of his lifestyle, and he learned how to anticipate the onset of an attack if he lapsed. He discovered that he was most vulnerable when his Control Pause was low and his breathing deep and found that a startling relief of his symptoms took place when he breathed shallowly. Not only did his Control Pause go up, but he felt very much better.

After two weeks Tony no longer needed Ventolin at all and could take four flights of stairs without pausing for breath. He had also realized that it was easy to incorporate Breath Connection exercises into his demanding business schedule and was well worth the small effort that it required.

Preparing for Breath Connection

• Learn how to check your pulse (see pages 53–55).

• Read and fully understand the theoretical parts of this book.

• Breathe through your nose and keep your mouth closed at all times, except when talking, eating, or drinking.

• If you are taking oral steroids now but are engaged in a plan to step down the intake, as described in an earlier chapter, stop doing so. From now on, keep your steroid intake at the same level until your asthma has improved to such a degree that we would describe it as mild and one puff of your bronchodilator is sufficient to alleviate your symptoms.

• Use bronchodilators only when you need to. Don't take them to prevent an attack, and ignore any previous schedule you may have been following.

• Stop using a nebulizer on a regular basis. Use it only if two or three puffs of the inhaler or other form of medication does not work. If you must use a nebulizer, try to limit use to 30 seconds—at the very maximum, no more than three minutes.

• Take only a single puff of your inhaler at any one time.

- Avoid long-lasting, slow-working bronchodilators such as Atrovent or Serevent because you will need faster relief than these can offer.

- Practice shallow breathing. Think of this as being the start of a training course and remember that bad, old habits always take time to unlearn, especially when you are striving to adopt new, good ones at the same time. Within five days there should be a clear improvement noticeable enough to encourage perseverance.

- Remember that dedicated retraining after a lifetime of incorrect breathing may actually take some weeks. This is a little like dieting. You may initially lose a great deal of weight, but you soon reach a plateau, and subsequent changes are less dramatic. Your weight loss may even be more difficult to maintain. Similarly, with the Breath Connection program, some severe asthmatics feel so elated by the immediate results of the first few days that they are discouraged when the dramatic rate of improvement is not maintained over the next stages. Try not to be discouraged. The essential groundwork had been laid and steady, permanent improvement will follow. We do not offer the respiratory equivalent of a crash diet, but we know that our spectacularly fast early results can inspire patients to maintain the discipline.

- You will have learned to try to use your lungs less. Make sure that the amplitude of your chest (full expansion) has been decreased and that the movement of your diaphragm has decreased.

- Remember to tape your mouth shut at night (see pages 51–52).

- Take time to read and follow the dietary guidelines we discuss in Chapter 12, which will enhance recovery.

- Remember never to push your Control Pause beyond the point of comfort, as it will aggravate the risk of hyperventilation.
- Never push your Control Pause above 60.

We cannot overstress the fact that the Breath Connection techniques can have a powerful effect—as powerful as any drugs—and care must be taken to follow the instructions exactly, in order to achieve maximum effect.

CHARLOTTE

Severe asthma can strike at any age. Charlotte was a late developer and did not experience symptoms until her late sixties. Each of the several doctors she consulted prescribed different drugs and she has, over time, absorbed a confusing amount of conflicting advice and information about asthma. Because she bruised easily and had concerns about osteoporosis and stomach problems—all common side effects of steroids—she took only one oral steroid a day. She was unaware that during hospital visits she had been given large doses of steroids. Because many patients are alarmed by the use of steroids, doctors and nurses in hospitals often refer to them euphemistically. For this reason, Charlotte had no reason to believe that she was being given a high dose of a medication that she did not want.

Manufactured steroids can have side effects, but can be useful as a temporary measure on the Breath Connection program. They can help to rebalance the breathing while you retrain. After a short time, the dosage can be reduced under supervision, and your body will begin to produce its own natural steroids.

Having read about us, Charlotte flew from her home in North America to take part in a Breath Connection workshop in London. She claimed that talking helped her to breathe, and she was not at all sure that keeping her mouth closed would work. But she listened and learned and was determined to follow the Breath Connection regime to the letter. We explained to her that properly prescribed steroids have their uses for asthmatics and indeed may well have saved her life on several occasions in the past.

Charlotte found that after one session—which she had not enjoyed in the least!—she could sleep peacefully at night. After three months of faithfully following Breath Connection exercises, Charlotte's asthma had become so mild that she could go for weeks without needing to take more than the occasional puff on a ventilator. Her medication was now just 5 percent of what it was when she came to see us. Only occasionally, to ward off colds or flu, Charlotte takes between half and one tablet of Prednisone. Her hospital visits are now a thing of the past.

The Technique

1. Check your Control Pause and your pulse (see pages 48 and 53–55).
2. Practice shallow breathing (see page 50).
3. Continue to take your pulse, then do the Control Pause and afterward decrease your breathing for two minutes.
4. Do another Control Pause, relax for a few minutes, and then breathe lightly. You may feel slightly heady, but this is perfectly normal and nothing to worry about. You're just experiencing the power of the

Breath Connection techniques and in these early days some sensations may feel strange.

5. Do another Control Pause followed by four minutes of shallow breathing.

6. Do another Control Pause. Rest for a few minutes.

7. Do the Control Pause again but this time shallow breathe for six minutes afterward.

8. Check your Control Pause and take a rest.

9. Check your Control Pause again and this time shallow breathe for eight minutes. Repeat number 6 above.

10. Now do the Control Pause exercise once again, followed by 10 minutes of shallow breathing. Check your CP again and then take your pulse.

The entire exercise should take only about 25 minutes.

As you go through each stage of the CP and pulse checking (see pages 244–245), make a note of the figures. When you study them later, you will see that as the Control Pause figure went up, the pulse rate came down. You will certainly feel better after completing this exercise and should get into the habit of performing it regularly and charting progress so that you can see, week by week, how you have progressed.

Carry on three times a day, two hours before meals, for three or four weeks or until you no longer need to resort to bronchodilators. Stay on your steroids. These should only be reduced under the guidance of a Breath Connection practitioner or a sympathetic doctor.

Some people worry that their GP will be hostile or cynical to the Breath Connection program and it is true that a few of them might be dismissive. If you encounter resistance from your GP, I suggest that you show him or her this book.

Daily technique for overcoming severe asthma

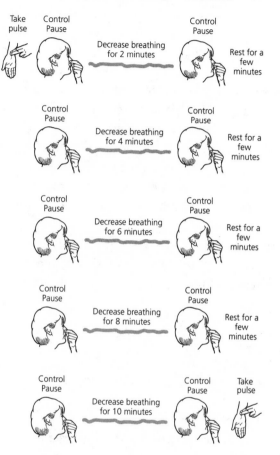

The Breath Connection technique has been associated with Australian research of the highest repute, and your doctor will be more likely to respond to the project if he or she is aware of its authenticity. If your doctor steadfastly refuses to help you to progress via the Breath Connection program, you can, of course, always ask for a second opinion.

If you do not feel any better after a month or so, you may need some individual coaching from a Breath Connection practitioner. Courses are available all over the United Kingdom and the United States. If there isn't a course in your area, you may want to combine a holiday or a business trip with a visit to one of our centers. Above all, don't be discouraged. Failure to respond to the Breath Connection techniques outlined here simply means that you have very individual needs, and they will need to be assessed and dealt with by an expert. We are confident that the technique will work for you, even if it does take more time. Self-help isn't always possible, particularly when a condition is deep rooted.

In the course of following the previously described steps for a few weeks, you might still experience an asthma attack. If so, you will find the following advice helpful.

Overcoming a Severe Asthma Attack

Whenever you experience the onset of an attack, stop whatever you are doing. Then take the following steps:

1. Take your pulse and do a Control Pause.
2. Then shallow breathe for 10 minutes and take another Control Pause.
3. Take your pulse again.
4. If this doesn't work, Professor Buteyko recommends that you take just one puff from your inhaler. Then, if necessary, take another puff five minutes later.
5. If you're still in discomfort, use your nebulizer for one to three minutes. Only if this fails should you use the full nebulizer. The most important thing is that you

allow your body the chance to muster its own resistance before leaning on your familiar props.

Professor Buteyko also points out that if your puffer didn't work, you might need to increase your oral steroids—in consultation with your doctor—because it suggests that your asthma is unstable. In some cases, you may be able to decrease your oral steroids, with your doctor's advice, but only gradually and under the following conditions:

- You don't use your inhaler more than three to four times a day.
- Your control pause is not less than 10 seconds.
- Your pulse is not more than 100 beats per minute.
- Your attacks haven't been sharp or sudden.

This technique for severe asthmatics is a first step toward conquering asthma completely. Steroid use and requirements will vary between individuals and it is impossible to formulate a system that will work for everyone. You will need to work fairly closely with your doctor, and, perhaps, a Breath Connection practitioner to assess your needs on a weekly basis, until the condition has been righted.

Technique for dealing with a severe asthma attack

Take pulse   Control Pause   Shallow breathe for 10 minutes   Control Pause   Take pulse

Diary of a Severe Asthmatic

The following diary gives you an example of what a severe asthmatic might expect during five days on the Breath Connection program. Once again, responses will differ between individuals, and different people will benefit in different ways. Every person will also progress at his or her own pace, so don't be alarmed if your progress is unlike what we describe here.

Day One
The severe asthmatic will continue to take steroid medication but will be able to restrict use of puffers and other forms of relief and will usually be able to set aside nebulizers. Quality of sleep will improve and there will be far fewer problems in the early morning.

Day Two
Breath control will have improved and there will be even less need for puffers. Breathlessness will be reduced and appropriate eating patterns for both the underweight and overweight will begin to emerge.

Day Three
There will be a marked improvement in the Control Pause and all other general symptoms. Your overall condition will have improved. There will be further reduction in the need for drugs.

Day Four
This steady improvement in all areas will intensify.

Day Five

Changes will inspire all-around confidence, and you will find it easier to complete the exercises. You will be able to keep your mouth closed without too much conscious effort.

After a few weeks there will be a reduction in your need for medication of about 50 percent, considerable improvement in the Control Pause, and you will be able to endure colds and flu without an automatic trip to the hospital. Asthma attacks and symptoms will have become mild and a single puff on a reliever will be enough to stave off an attack. The quality of your life will have improved enormously, and simple things that nonasthmatics take for granted, such as walking down the street without breathlessness, will become the norm. Coughing fits will be eliminated or greatly shortened, and your weight will have become more balanced—or, at least, well on the way to becoming so. You'll be sleeping much more peacefully, which means that you will function better in every single aspect of your professional and private life.

Key Points to Remember
- Sleep on your left side (see page 52).
- Tape up your mouth (see page 51) before sleep and whenever you are home alone.
- Avoid protein meals in the evening (see page 193), which can take a great deal of oxygen to digest and increase the possibility of suffering an asthma attack in the night or following morning.
- Avoid all dairy foods, which can increase mucus production.

7

Breath Connection for Emphysema and Bronchitis

Emphysema is slow suffocation.

Because it is generally believed that cigarette smoking has intensified, if not caused, the condition, many sufferers will have to endure the unsympathetic attitudes of others who believe that they have only themselves to blame. This can cause feelings of isolation and depression in the sufferer, which can make the condition worse. Asthmatics are, at least, spared the lack of sympathy and indignity of being told that they are the cause of their own illness.

The horrific symptoms of emphysema outweigh the severity of the crime, and no sufferer should be treated with disdain. Emphysema is a frightening, serious illness, and it can take a dramatic course that leaves the sufferer literally gasping for breath on a daily basis.

Naturally, we do advise against cigarette smoking, which is a dangerous habit. Hostile warnings are, however, unlikely to change the habits of a committed smoker and illness should garner sympathy, whatever its cause. Even more controversially, perhaps, we are not convinced that smoking is the cause of emphysema. We do know that emphysemics who smoke will feel markedly better if they follow the Breath Connection program.

The most punishing and cruel aspect of emphysema is the fact that it completely restricts the life of the sufferer. Not only do emphysemics suffer debilitating breathlessness but they experience a crippling reduction in mobility that makes it harder and harder for them to lead a normal life. If you are emphysemic and already struggling with physical restrictions, the Breath Connection program can help to arrest many of your symptoms. If your illness is in its early stages, we can help you to avoid, or certainly delay, the worst symptoms if you start to follow our program now. A normal life, or at least a semblance of one, can be resumed and your life expectancy can be increased.

You will need to set aside some time to follow the Breath Connection program and self-discipline will be required. The chances are that family and friends, anxious about your condition, will do all they can to encourage you and they will be almost as gratified as you will be to observe the improvement in your condition. Every step toward restored mobility can lead to another and then another.

MARIE

Marie was on the waiting list for a double lung transplant, although she had little confidence that even this drastic measure would help her much. At 74, she had severe emphysema and had been confined to a wheelchair for several years. Her massive daily medication included six to eight nebulizers, with up to 25 puffs of Ventolin between doses. She also inhaled steroids (the incredibly powerful Beclomethasone) twice a day and often took oral steroids as well. Moreover, Marie took antibiotics whenever she had a chest infection. While she was waiting for a hospital place, Marie was given courage by her husband to start the Breath Connection program. Because she had been attached to an oxygen supply 24 hours a day, she was, understandably, fearful about taking the pipes out of her nose to do the Control Pause.

Marie used to be a smoker, and although she had stopped some 20 years earlier, she had been told that smoking was the cause of her illness. Her face was ashen, a reflection of the very low oxygen level in her blood, and she often had to sleep in her wheelchair, which meant that she got little proper rest. Rising from it to go to the bathroom at night was a regular nightmare. In short, Marie's life was desperately restricted.

She embarked upon Breath Connection after she had been waiting for her operation for almost a year. She took almost immediate heart when she learned from her Breath Connection practitioner that surgery would probably be unnecessary if she undertook the program. She was also surprised to learn that he did not consider that her old smoking habit was the cause of her current condition.

Her first Control Pause was very low—only five seconds—but after just a few exercises on her first day, she only needed to be attached to her oxygen supply for three hours a day and to use only two nebulizers. On the second day, she only used the nebulizer once, in the morning, and had one oxygen boost in the evening. On day three, she was able to rise from her wheelchair and take some faltering steps. After years in a wheelchair, her leg muscles had atrophied, but this would soon be remedied.

Her Breath Connection practitioner told her to count the number of steps she was able to take every day to see how they increased. She was also advised to shallow breathe upon waking each morning. She was to eat only when she was hungry, which was a considerable challenge for Marie, who had become used to eating heartily five times a day.

By the fifth day of the program, Marie was not using a nebulizer, was down to two or three puffs of Ventolin, and could begin to walk 50 meters four or five times a day. After another five days, she could double that distance and her skin was healthily pink. Three months later, Marie met her GP when she was out shopping—on her feet. His surprise at the sight of her was such that he rather tactlessly told her that, because he hadn't seen her for some time, he had assumed she was dead. Marie was far from dead.

In the past, there was very little hope for emphysemics. Breath Connection can change that. You can work from home as well as with a practitioner and witness steady progress. Carefully document your progress on the charts on pages 246 or 247, and over time you will see results. Initially, results may be slight and sluggish, but continued effort will bring permanent change and the vise of emphysema can first be loosened and then reversed to a significant degree.

Emphysema is a severe respiratory disorder wherein the air sacs (alveoli) in the lungs are permanently enlarged and partially damaged. Lung tissue is usually hardened and rendered inflexible by the loss of blood to essential vessels that nurture this tissue. Lung capacity is decreased and patients experience shortness of breath, especially when walking uphill or even upstairs. Many emphysemics need to use oxygen at night and some have to sit in a wheelchair attached to an oxygen cylinder.

But, until doctors accept that the major cause of emphysema is not smoking, and that double lung transplants are not the only answer, the majority of cases will never be successfully treated.

Emphysema Myths

The facts are complicated and may seem to be contradictory:

• The majority of emphysema patients stopped smoking long before they contracted the illness; indeed, in some cases 20 years have elapsed since the last cigarette, and some patients, including many children, have never smoked at all.

• Most doctors will say that asthma and emphysema are two very different conditions, and yet they prescribe the same drugs to both groups, often in larger amounts to the emphysemics. All emphysemics hyperventilate, in fact, they overbreathe more than asthmatics. Yet doctors continue to tell them that they should breathe more deeply.

• We know that emphysemics breathe somewhere between three and five times the norm, and that this advice is compounding the problem.

• Doctors often prescribe oxygen for emphysema. However, the air we breathe contains 21 percent oxygen, already more than our bodies need. People who live in high altitudes, where oxygen levels are lower, tend to live longer, stronger lives than those at lower elevations, and yet doctors continue to prescribe 100 percent oxygen which is known to be harmful, even toxic.

Not Just a Lung Disorder

The conventional medical profession tends to view emphysema as being simply a lung or breathing problem. Their answer is to replace the faulty part with a new one, much like a car manufacturer would replace a faulty part in an engine that isn't working properly. This is completely at odds with the way we see things at The Hale Clinic. We believe that all conditions should be treated holistically—that is, addressing the mind and the whole body. When one part of the body goes wrong, it is usually a reflection that there is an imbalance in the body, not just in that one part. Going back to the example of the car manufacturer, we would recommend an entire service, not just a replacement part when the engine does not work properly. We believe that all systems are interactive.

Therefore, transplanting lungs in emphysemics is not the answer. The root imbalance will still exist within the body, and a seriously ill person will have the additional trauma of a serious operation. So often emphysema patients remain stricken with disability even after such costly surgery, and there is, of course, a risk of complete failure, as there is with any operation.

The fact is that Professor Buteyko was right when he discovered that emphysema is one of the body's mechanisms to fight hyperventilation. He found that the body reduces lung capacity in order to limit its loss of carbon dioxide and will increase it again when a balanced and quieter breathing pattern is reestablished.

By using the Breath Connection self-care program, emphysema sufferers have found that the advance of their condition has been slowed down or halted, that they have been easily able to reduce their drug intake—both bronchodilators and steroids—and thereby minimizing previous drug-related side effects. Every aspect of their quality of life has improved, from sleep and emotional state of mind to the ability to participate in normal activities such as walking and playing with children and grandchildren. Very often, working under specialist guidance, their visible improvements are so obvious that any previous threat of a lung transplant has been consigned to history.

As always we advise you to undertake our program with care and in consultation with your doctor or under the guidance of a Breath Connection practitioner. Those suffering from emphysema or other bronchial disorders should not undertake self-care, if you are prone to any of the related conditions noted in Appendix B. The extra support and supervision you will receive from an expert can only hasten your recovery.

Mild and Severe Emphysema

Preparing for Breath Connection

- It is essential that emphysemics strive toward a healthy lifestyle that includes physical exercise. For milder conditions, this means walking, swimming, cycling, horseriding, or jogging every day, always with a closed mouth, however great the exertion may seem.

- The most important thing is to enjoy your physical movement—however limited it may be in the beginning—and to remember that by taking on these activities, you are helping yourself to reduce medication, as well as to feel better.

- Emphysemics take two types of drug: steroids—either inhaled or in tablet form—and puffers, Salbutamol, Ventolin, Serevent, and nebulizers. Breathing exercises are essential for their efficacy.

Daily technique for mild to severe emphysema

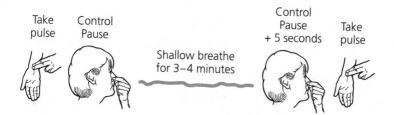

Each morning before breakfast, before dinner and an hour before going to sleep do a Control Pause and then shallow breathe for three or four minutes. Then do another Control Pause with an extra five seconds. Charting your progress on a daily and week-by-week basis will help you to monitor your improvement.

Walking Exercises for Moderate to Severe Emphysema

1. For those with moderate to severe emphysema the first thing to learn is how to control your breath while walking. Sit comfortably, check your pulse, do a Control Pause, and begin to shallow breathe.

2. Now stand up and continue to shallow breathe very slowly, listening to your breathing. Begin to take a few steps, walking very carefully round the room for about 20 to 25 paces. You should try and clear your mind of any thoughts so that you are completely relaxed. These exercises are often best practiced somewhere safely familiar such as in your own home.

3. Your breathing now will be deeper than it was when you were sitting down and this is quite normal. You

should feel that your breathing is absolutely under your control.

If you become breathless, feel you are losing control, and have a desire to open your mouth you can do the following:

- Keep walking and try to suppress your overbreathing by attempting to take in less air with each intake of breath.
- Slow down and walk even more slowly.
- Stop, hold your breath, and begin to walk very slowly again.

Your ability to walk without becoming breathless, while keeping your mouth closed, depends on the Control Pause. If this is very low, walking even a few meters will be beyond you. But if you can increase your Control Pause to 40 or 45 seconds you will be able to run—yes, run—upstairs to the third floor without distress.

You should now rest to take your breathing rate down. Then you can start again, walking a little faster this time. Soon, you should be able to walk at the rate of the average person in the street.

Each time, walk for as long as you can, but plan a realistic distance that will not cause you to slow down or to lose control of your breathing. Try 20 meters on first day, gradually increasing to 50 meters by the end of the week. When you're up to 5 kilometers a day, you've reached your goal. It's a great achievement! Not all physically fit people are able to walk that far without effort. Some emphysemics even find that they get so used to the swing of walking quite briskly that they have trouble walking slowly!

The important thing to remember is to keep your mouth closed at all times, whatever your walking speed. Some people find this quite a challenge and say that it increases their breathlessness. You will need to find your own correct pace—the one at which walking and breathing is comfortable and possible without opening the mouth. You might be ambling or positively striding—find what is the right speed for you. The point of this technique is to retrain your breathing; the other benefits of the physical exercise are secondary. Once you have learned to control your breathing, you may want to go on to more challenging activities such as sports, cycling, or going to the gym. If you still find it difficult to keep your mouth closed while taking any form of exercise, keep it shut with tape.

Once again the micropore tape we recommend is light and barely visible: it's not like placing a strip of masking tape across your mouth! If you do feel self-conscious about it, consider that many cyclists and even pedestrians in cities wear masks against pollution. You'll be wearing an adapted form!

So, to remind you

- Do your Control Pause three times a day, before breakfast, lunch, and dinner.
- Shallow breathe for three or four minutes between CPs and add five seconds to the second Control Pause of each session before taking your pulse.
- Don't forget to record your progress on the chart!

Sitting Exercises for Severe Emphysema

If your emphysema is so severe that you are in a wheelchair and attached to an oxygen balloon for long periods, it's obvious that you will not be able to engage in the walking program previously outlined. But being wheelchair-bound doesn't mean that you can't recondition your breathing and make some small physical movements.

Unless you are completely paralyzed, you can work on your breath and retrain your lung muscles. Don't assume that your need for a wheelchair will be infinite. More importantly, don't use it as an excuse. There is no reason why you can't fight to lessen your disabilities. By following the exercises we recommend in the next section, you really have nothing to lose!

As usual, the exercises should be completed at least two hours before mealtimes and an hour before going to bed.

The Technique

Exercise A

1. Control your breathing by taking slow, shallow breaths through the nose. Take off your oxygen straw—don't worry, you will be fine.
2. Check your pulse and measure your Control Pause. Now breathe out gently.
3. Then hold your breath out and at the same time tense the muscles of your hands for up to three seconds.
4. Then relax, breathe in gently, and continue to shallow breathe for a few minutes until you are ready for the next exercise. Keep your mouth closed.

Exercise B

1. Breathe out, hold your breath, and tense the muscles in your legs for up to four seconds.
2. Relax, breathe in gently, and continue to shallow breathe through the nose—as always—for three or four minutes.

Exercise C

1. Breathe out, hold your breath out, and this time tense your whole body for three seconds.
2. Relax, breathe in gently, and continue to shallow breathe for four or five minutes, mouth closed.

Repeat these three exercises as often as you can, always checking your Control Pause before and afterward. Your CP should improve by a second or two each time, your pulse rate will be reduced, and your body will feel warmer afterward. When you have completed each session, replace your oxygen straw only if you feel you must. If you think you can manage without it for some of the day, try to do so. But put the straw back on before going to sleep.

It is particularly important for emphysemics not to push the Control Pause too high. Your body's instincts will be the best monitor here. If you begin to feel uncomfortable during the Control Pause, stop and begin to shallow breathe for a few minutes. Look upon the Breath Connection program as something to be administered in dosages just as you would regard medication prescribed by your doctor. You should never exceed your Control Pause beyond comfortable limits unless you are taking guidance from a Breath Connection practitioner.

Regardless of the severity of your condition as an emphysemic, this is a summary of the basic guidelines:

- Sleep on your left side (see page 52).
- Keep your mouth closed as often as possible.
- Tape your mouth when sleeping or during the day, if alone.
- Avoid dairy foods such as milk, cheese, and yogurt, which can increase mucus buildup, and cut down on

protein, which increases your need for oxygen. Do not eat a protein meal in the evening.

Breath Connection for Bronchitis

Bronchitis may not be as serious a disorder as asthma or emphysema but it can, nonetheless, generate enormous distress and create restrictions in the lives of its victims. It is another condition predicated by a shortage of carbon dioxide and exacerbated by overbreathing.

For those who suffer from it, perhaps the most troubling aspect of this illness is the continual, painful, chest-wracking cough that it brings and, if not properly treated, bronchitis can easily lead to those other, more severe, respiratory disorders. So, bronchitis should never be seen as some relatively minor, seasonal, or merely inconvenient illness. We take it very seriously indeed and regard it as a very unpleasant but useful early warning that the health has begun a dangerous downward spiral. Action now can save all sufferers a future of even more debilitating disease.

Medical reference books define *bronchitis* as an "inflammation of the mucous membrane of the bronchi (the two main airways to the lungs) which often affects the throat, larynx and bronchioles." Chronic bronchitis is normally associated with swelling of the bronchial mucous glands, which are irritated by cigarettes and air pollution. Despite much current thinking, we know that these may be factors in the exacerbation of the condition, but they are not the root cause. The variable and frequently damp climate in Britain has also been held responsible for a number of cases.

It is also commonly believed that bronchitis is caused by infection, like sore throats, head colds, and pneumonia, as it is usually preceded by the sort of bugs that spread rapidly around air-conditioned offices and centrally heated houses. These render us vulnerable to attack from microorganisms which settle in the sinuses and strain our defense mechanisms. Certainly much bronchitis begins this way, but one of the reasons why it becomes a chronic, rather than short-term, condition is the fact that our immune systems are not strong enough to fight infections—and that is often the result of improper breathing. Most smokers never suffer from bronchitis. Yet many people who have never smoked in their lives do develop this disorder. The polluted air in the cities where some of us live can't be the cause; bronchitis afflicts many people who live in clean environments. Smoking and air pollution can exacerbate the problem, but they don't cause it. The cause of bronchitis—like so many other respiratory conditions—remains a mystery.

JAMES

James had chronic bronchitis and he was only seven years old. His father brought the boy to us because he had endured violent coughing fits for nine months and nothing—conventional medicine, a recent course of Chinese herbs, trips to the seaside and mountains—had helped. James's father had been outraged when the family GP suggested that the boy was secretly smoking, and his disillusionment led him to Breath Connection.

When we first met James, he had tonsillitis as well, the most recent of a string of illnesses and infections that had kept him away from school for long periods of time. On only the second day at Breath Connection, James's cough stopped. Over the next five months, having learned to practice the Breath Connection exercises at home, James did not suffer from any colds or flu. His personal best!

Antibiotics can sometimes help in cases of pneumonia, but only if the pneumonia is bacterial. All doctors admit that antibiotics are useless against viruses of any type, and many cases of pneumonia are viral. To date, all attempts by scientists to identify the microorganisms that settle in the bronchi—causing bronchitis and pneumonia, and proving resilient to the efforts of the immune system to fight them off—have failed. The few microorganisms that have been pinpointed appear to be carried by the majority of us, and yet few of us go on to contract the illnesses. Whatever bug is killing us has continued to elude scientists, as is the reason why some people have the capacity to fight it, and others do not.

Perhaps even more importantly, there is no cure for bronchitis, because its cause is unknown. Like asthma, bronchitis is usually treated with drugs to ease or mask the symptoms.

Hyperventilation and Bronchitis

Professor Buteyko has long maintained that hyperventilation affects the metabolic responses of every cell in the body, starting with the nervous system, then affecting the heart, and third, targeting the lungs and bronchi. He has said that when the cells of the bronchial "tree" become damaged, inflammation and swelling occur in the upper part. What we call bronchitis will follow. When the problems affect the lower part of the tree, there is danger of a severe condition known as *bronchioectathis*. This is very difficult to treat.

Any infection, adverse weather condition, cigarette smoke, or even something as innocent as eating ice cream can aggravate this condition. It is also known that it often precipitates asthma, which is yet another reason why we should study it and strive to unravel its mysteries. These two conditions are clearly linked in that patients with a characteristic bronchial cough may suddenly experience breathing difficulty, develop a bronchospasm, and become what is called asthmatic. The correct term should be *asthma with bronchitis*. As Professor Buteyko has explained, when patients begin to develop a pattern of hyperventilation, they lose carbon dioxide. This upsets the metabolic balance of the bronchial cells as they become further inflamed and weakened. By increasing breath intake and further upsetting the oxygen/carbon dioxide mix, the body implements its reserve defense mechanism—a bronchospasm—and the terrible coughing begins.

Fortunately, not everyone with bronchitis will go on to develop asthma. For this to happen, there must first be a predisposition to bronchospasm. People without adequate natural immunity may develop emphysema, or bronchioectathis, which can be far worse. Yet there are others who have stronger defense mechanisms who will suffer bronchial spasm at times, but never develop bronchitis. Asthmatics—in particular, children—may develop bronchitis as well, mainly due to the use of certain inhalants. People who are concerned about wheezing may visit a doctor who has no real way of determining whether he or she should be treating asthma or bronchitis! The truth is that almost no one in authority knows what to do.

Until about 40 years ago, it was common to call such attacks in young children "wheezy bronchitis" or "bronchitis with phlegm," as the word *asthma* was considered to be too frightening. But, at some stage, doctors began to believe that all children thus afflicted were indeed asthmatic, and they prescribed treatment accordingly. Asthma treatments were often mistakenly and heavily prescribed, causing damage to sufferers who did not need them.

If you suffer from bronchitis, we strongly recommend that you follow the Breath Connection technique for bronchitis. A few simple exercises every day will scarcely inconvenience you, yet they could spare you the threat of much worse things to come, as your breathing is rebalanced and your bronchitis recedes. As soon as you see your Control Pause rising on your daily chart you will know that the downward spiral toward serious disease has been arrested.

Please never optimistically assume that because you have a disorder that you can live with, no serious action needs to be taken. Severe, chronic ill health sometimes starts with signals too slight or minor to be registered. Perhaps, therefore, we should be grateful for the unmistakable ways in which bronchitis announces itself. Indeed, all pain could be looked at it in this way—it is a clear warning from our bodies that something is not right. Our bodies are telling us to take action now, before it is too late.

Daily technique for bronchitis

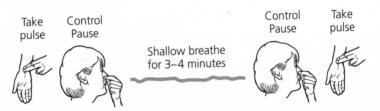

Repeat this exercise in the morning before breakfast and before you go to bed at night. Monitor your daily progress in the charts for the Weekly Bronchitis Program.

This type of analogy applies to a smoker who ignores a light but persistent cough and thus the stealthy development of lung cancer, or the person with an acute toothache who puts off going to the dentist until it is too late to rescue the tooth. Listen to your body; don't ignore its messages.

It is, naturally, human nature to hope or assume that a problem will go away. Our bodies are far too precious to risk such an optimistic attitude, and we should seek advice at the first sign of something being amiss. It may be an overused cliché, but there is no doubt that prevention is far better than a cure.

Chronic illness is expensive—both personally, and to the taxpayer—and can, in some cases, be very difficult to treat. The longer you leave a health condition, the longer it will take to cure. If you discovered some evidence of dry rot in your home, would you wait until the problem became more extensive before seeking help? Not likely. You'd be worried and possibly annoyed about the expense and nuisance of getting it fixed, but you would be aware that the problem could become worse if you didn't treat it now. Your health is more important than your house—make sure you give it at least the same care. This is why we take illnesses such as bronchitis—and others mentioned in a later chapter—very seriously.

Let's look at the four principal bronchial situations and combinations and consider how to deal with them:

- Bronchitis
- Bronchitis and mild asthma
- Bronchitis and severe asthma
- Bronchitis and emphysema

Typical of the first situation is a cough which can be defined as pure hyperventilation, or overbreathing. But we must not assume that this is just a case of simple bronchitis. There is a very strong chance that other illnesses will emerge and develop in this weakened area of the body. The consistent coughing will have reduced carbon dioxide levels throughout the whole body, and all parts will have been affected. Defense mechanisms, such as asthma, bronchospasm, or the production of excess mucus, will also be evident. Other dangers are pulmonary sclerosis (a hardening of the lung tissue) or fibrosis (the function of the lung is affected when fibrous matter builds up), which can be very serious indeed. Bronchitis can also lead to heart disease, high blood pressure, and a whole host of other conditions stemming from hyperventilation. There is no such thing as "simple" bronchitis.

This chain can be broken, and the first step is to eradicate the bronchitis, so that the danger of other conditions, many of them potentially fatal, is reduced. Throughout this book we are aiming to prove that you have not been saddled with a disease that is unmanageable or irreversible. We can empower you to overcome physical disabilities that can be righted and we urge you to persevere. Take preventive action now, and you can avoid unnecessarily ill health for as long as you live. We are pleased to note that more and more people are seeing a persistent cough as evidence of a problem, rather than just suppressing it with cough medicines or, worse, ignoring it completely. This action could save their lives.

The Anti-Coughing Technique

There is not a finite amount of mucus in your bronchial tubes, as many people imagine. You can cough for days, or months, or years on end, and your body will still continue to produce mucus, and there will always be something to cough up. The production of mucus is one of your body's defense mechanisms against the loss of carbon dioxide, and mucus is replenished as quickly as it is lost.

Preventing your body from producing too much mucus will stop your cough.

In the grip of an exhausting cough—a common and distressing occurrence for those with bronchitis, asthma, and emphysema—the untrained impulse is to clear your lungs of the mucus that has built up. This sensation is particularly noticeable in the morning. Coughing is the body's natural response to mucus buildup and it is yet another defense mechanism, designed to expel foreign bodies and anything else hampering the breathing process. But these are not normal circumstances. You must learn to resist the urge to cough. Instead, you must learn to control the hyperventilation that has caused the buildup of mucus, and the spasm, in the first place. Medication might help, but not as much as the steps on page 120).

We know that the cough is caused by the damage that hyperventilation has created in the lining of your bronchi. We also know that a spasm of coughing will cause you to overbreathe even more. Coughing spasms can be lengthy and exhausting. Occasionally resorting to a simple over-the-counter cough suppressant may be helpful, but there are more natural means. The anti-cough technique will always bring relief, and you may also be able to avoid coughing spasms entirely by strengthening your immunity to bronchitis. The daily self-care program, which incorporates the Control Pause, will help you do so.

Anti-coughing technique

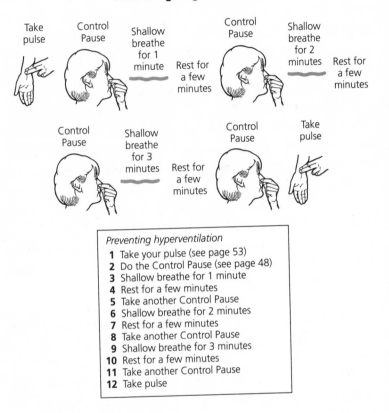

Preventing hyperventilation
1 Take your pulse (see page 53)
2 Do the Control Pause (see page 48)
3 Shallow breathe for 1 minute
4 Rest for a few minutes
5 Take another Control Pause
6 Shallow breathe for 2 minutes
7 Rest for a few minutes
8 Take another Control Pause
9 Shallow breathe for 3 minutes
10 Rest for a few minutes
11 Take another Control Pause
12 Take pulse

If you have bronchitis with mild asthma, you can also follow the technique offered on page 79. This technique is useful for asthma symptoms, including coughing.

Bronchitis and severe asthma are the most difficult to treat, and this type of bronchitis must be taken very seriously. Use the anti-coughing technique and refer to the program for severe asthmatics on page 95.

Bronchitis with emphysema is, unhappily, a typical combination. Emphysemics often feel like coughing after the briefest of walks or conversations. This problem takes some time to treat, but it is worth the investment. Start by practicing the anti-coughing technique. Refer also to the sections earlier in this chapter on dealing with emphysema.

You may think that the time spent attempting to relieve a cough is wasteful. We assure you that it is well worth your while. Think of the time and energy spent struggling through coughing fits. Think how they might have impaired your work or affected your colleagues' work. Make this technique a priority, even if it means getting up a little earlier or turning up at work a little bit late.

Use the Anti-Coughing Technique (AT) at the first sign of a cough. It is often easier to stop an asthma attack than it is to arrest and gain control of a coughing fit. In the case of asthma you can always reach for medication, but nothing, except this technique, will stop your coughing. Be patient. Eventually you will be in control.

For existing mucus, you way wonder whether it is better to cough it up or swallow it. We suggest coughing it out, but only when it is comfortable for you to do so. Don't force it, and never use expectorants or any other cough medicines, including herbal remedies, when participating in the Breath Connection program. Try to release your mucus in a single, easy motion, or you will risk further hyperventilation and overbreathing.

8

Breath Connection for Panic Attacks and Stress

Thousands of people who would not describe themselves as being asthmatic endure frightening panic attacks without realizing that hyperventilation—the same cause of asthma—is at the root of their condition. Panic attacks can be incredibly debilitating, and because there is no instant remedy in the form of an inhaler as there is during an asthma attack, it can be even more frightening. Conventional doctors tend to regard panic attacks as brief and physiologically normal responses to stressful situations, and they are largely regarded as being harmless.

Stressful situations can, of course, induce an attack, and an attack is most certainly a natural response by the body to fear or panic. However, for some people, normal, everyday activities can cause an attack. Shopping, using public transportation, taking an elevator, or even just walking into a party can trigger an alarming series of physical responses. Moreover, the fear of an attack can generate serious, deeper psychological debility.

During a panic attack, there may be dizziness, palpitations, chest constriction, and muscle fatigue. For some there are blackouts, a feeling of near suffocation, and even a fear of a heart attack. The attack may pass quickly, and some sufferers may be able to calm themselves by constantly reassuring themselves that they will be all right. But the fact is, the condition that caused the attack—hidden hyperventilation—remains even after the attack has passed. Permanent avoidance of panic attacks can be achieved by following the Breath Connection program.

The urge to take deep breaths at the onset of an attack can be overwhelming, and certainly in the past, doctors and psychologists recommended just that action. One established remedy has been to breathe into a paper bag, and then to inhale from it—a surprising confirmation that during hyperventilation our bodies need carbon dioxide, not great gulps of oxygen.

Counseling, abdominal breathing exercises, and relaxation techniques have often been suggested for the treatment of panic attacks. However, when we hyperventilate, the blood vessels throughout the body—including those feeding the brain and heart—are constricted, and the nervous system is affected. It is unlikely that soothing words, however well-learned, will be of much use to someone fighting for breath in the grip of a sudden attack.

This particular form of what is called hidden hyperventilation and the overbreathing which exists between attacks can be simply addressed by Breath Connection. It is important to realize that a foundation for a severe panic attack is being laid if shallow breathing is not practiced on a day-to-day basis (see exercise on p. 134). As we have said earlier, attacks of this nature are often more worrying and more difficult to deal with than the kind of spasm endured by known asthmatics, who will probably have some form of relief on hand.

Technique for panic attacks

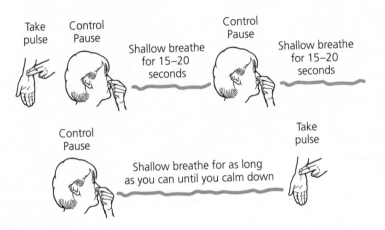

The Technique

1. If you are suffering a panic attack, stop and do the Control Pause three times. Shallow breathe for 15 to 20 seconds between each pause.

2. After the final Control Pause, shallow breathe for as long as you can manage or until you calm down. This can be anything from 5–60 minutes.

3. Do this before entering any situation in which fear might induce an attack, whether it is walking into a room full of strangers or simply facing a crowded street.

This exercise will boost your carbon dioxide level and stave off panic. However frightening it may seem, this sort of problem is normally a mild one. Gaining the confidence to know that you can overcome it will certainly help you to deal with other, more severe problems you may face.

If you cannot stop to practice this technique in the throes

of an attack, keep your mouth closed and try to shallow breathe through your nose.

Before embarking on the Breath Connection exercises in this chapter, you should ascertain whether you are suffering from any of the illnesses in Appendix B. If you do, it will be necessary for you to practice the Breath Connection program under the guidance of a qualified practitioner.

Stress

While panic can sometimes seem, and indeed may be, irrational, most of us have experienced stress and can understand the complicated chain of symptoms that accompany it. Demanding jobs, moving home, family life, relationships, financial problems, emotional pressure, and even joyful events such as Christmas, a wedding, childbirth, or a holiday can burden us with stress. For obvious reasons, divorce or bereavement can be even worse. Many people seek short-term relief with alcohol, nicotine, other drugs, or even food, but all of these can be avoided by following the Breath Connection program.

What Happens When We Are Stressed?

The stress reaction is a natural response to fear. It prepares the body for "fight or flight" by tensing the muscles and constricting the blood vessels. However, because most of the stressful experiences we encounter today do not require us to fight or flee, the body is left in a state of physical tension, which can result in a lowering of immunity, rendering us more susceptible to disease. There are literally dozens of common ailments associated with stress, including recurrent headaches, dizziness, rashes, colds and infections, panic attacks, aches and pains, loss of appetite, compulsive eating, irritability, fatigue, tearfulness, sleep problems, and lack of concentration. As you know from our earlier discussions, Breath Connection has been successful in helping almost all of these conditions. Most importantly, Breath Connection can help you to cope with stress in general.

The Technique

Try to control stress using the Control Pause technique (see page 48), in the following sequence, when you awake in the morning, before lunch, and before going to bed at night.

Daily technique for reducing stress generally

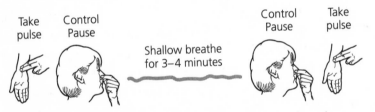

Take pulse   Control Pause   Shallow breathe for 3–4 minutes   Control Pause   Take pulse

Try this in the morning (before breakfast), before lunch, and before going to sleep.

If you are confronted with a potentially stressful situation at any other time of the day, a quick Control Pause and some shallow breathing will calm you down and enable you to deal with the situation more effectively. You can still rush to your meeting—only minutes later!

1. Do three Control Pauses, followed by 5-, 10- and then 15- or 20-second intervals.
2. Practice shallow breathing for two to three minutes.
3. Repeat if you do not feel calmer.

Calming technique for dealing with an immediate stressful situation

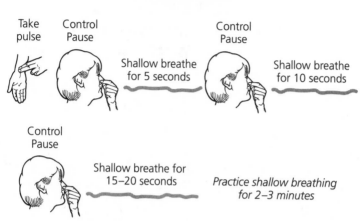

Take pulse

Control Pause

Shallow breathe for 5 seconds

Control Pause

Shallow breathe for 10 seconds

Control Pause

Shallow breathe for 15–20 seconds

Practice shallow breathing for 2–3 minutes

Meditation in the morning or at night can be enormously helpful, and we strongly recommend it. It is, however, seldom practical to meditate in the middle of a busy day. The preceding technique offers one of the best and fastest methods for stress relief that we know. We all live in a world and an environment complicated by choices that would have been unimaginable even to our parents' generation. Ever advancing technology does not, ironically, seem to have simplified our lives. But we can teach ourselves to adapt and cope with stresses and panics in the most natural way. Once again, you can breathe your problems away.

9

Holistic Self-Care for General Well-Being

We may appear to be healthy—with bright eyes, clear skin, shining hair, and strong limbs. We may play tennis or run, work hard all day yet still feel ready to go dancing all night. . . . How appealing the idea of perfect health is. A lucky few do have it—and, sadly, they are just a few! Luck it may seem, but in reality a good deal of subtle self-discipline may underpin that image of effortless total health.

Even if you are one of the lucky ones, don't become over-confident. However well you look, seem, and feel, you can fall prey to illness and it can come as a total shock. The best gymnasiums, cosmetic treatments, and the finest clothes may all contribute to a glorious illusion if, beneath the skin, something is going wrong. The increased stress of modern life, particularly in cities where no one can avoid breathing in toxic fumes, can take an insidious toll. The elimination system—that complex network which includes the kidneys, liver, and skin as well as the bowel itself—is put under a great deal of pressure in our society, with pollution, food additives and preservatives, increased alcohol intake and smoking, not to mention the number of chemicals that are used to grow even the freshest, healthiest-looking foods. We tend to brush off minor ailments as the result of being rundown or in need of a holiday. Even if we exercise and eat carefully, we can become ill.

Whether you feel healthy now, or suffer from common, niggling health problems, Breath Connection can make a huge difference in the way you look and feel—on and below the surface. Before you embark on a self-care program, check to ensure that you don't suffer from one of the illnesses listed in Appendix B.

DELIA

Delia had never been ill before she contracted a rare form of gland cancer. She was 45 years old. Her husband had been extremely supportive as she experimented with numerous alternative as well as conventional approaches to her disease. They even traveled to the Philippines, where they had read healers could perform miracles with cancer patients. Sadly, nothing worked for her. When Delia first came to us she could not walk to the second floor of our clinic. She was barely sleeping, her hair had all but dropped out, and she was so stressed and emotional that she was constantly tearful. Her tumor, she had been told, was the size of a fist. As well as affecting her hair, the chemotherapy and radiation had made Delia look like a woman of 60 instead of one in her prime.

After three months of working with Breath Connection on a special anticancer program Delia's tumor vanished. She regained her appetite and energy and slept well again. Soon she was ready to enjoy a proper holiday. Her previous doctors could only say that they must have been mistaken in their earlier diagnosis.

Tragically, two years later, when she was still feeling fit and well, and perhaps against her better judgment, she was persuaded to undergo a different course of treatment and she died soon afterward.

In almost all cases of cancer, patients are already in terminal stages of their illness when they come to us. However, the Breath Connection program can extend their lives by up to two years and also enhance the quality of that remaining time. All Breath Connection practitioners wish that patients would seek to recondition their breathing much sooner and thus reduce the danger of serious illness taking a fatal grip.

Monitoring Your Health

The importance of regularly monitoring your state of health via the Breath Connection program cannot be overstated. It will reflect the actual state of your health (which may differ from how well you think you are). If your Control Pause (see page 48) drops suddenly, you have been given a very clear signal that preventative measures are required. If you suspect this change might be stress-related, turn at once to the program for stress on page 125. The importance of this monitoring system cannot be overstated. You can put to rest any fears that terrible illness might be lurking round the corner by changing and maintaining your Control Pause. Checked regularly, it is an extremely accurate guide to your physical condition. If your Control Pause reaches and remains at 50 or 60, you will not suffer from degenerative disease. It's that simple.

This might seem like a very bold assertion, but it is based on Professor Buteyko's research in Russia involving literally millions of cases. He found that no single person with a CP of 50 to 60 had degenerative illness. This statistic, based on years of research, is enormously reassuring.

But our self-care program is not just about prevention. It has been devised to help well people to improve their health further, which will allow them to get even more out of life.

With a 50 to 60 Control Pause, all of your body systems—immune, hormonal, digestive, elimination, respiratory, cardiovascular, and the others—will be functioning properly. You will have more energy, need less sleep, and find your natural weight. The glowing good looks that often accompany such a state are a happy bonus. By following our program, your health will no longer be a vague area of mystery, confusion, and contradiction but something that you understand and experience, and it is measurable!

What Your Control Pause Tells You

Most people have long been aware that exercise and a well-balanced diet—with plenty of fresh fruit and vegetables and clean water—make a huge difference to health and well-being. But we are only just beginning to understand how incorrect breathing can negate the benefits of other sensible habits. If you find that your Control Pause is lower than 50, you should correct things by following the basic Breath Connection program. If—to your surprise and alarm—it is down toward 20, you should start immediate preventative measures to avert the risk of some form of degenerative disease taking hold later.

If you find you have a low Control Pause, don't panic. The problem will probably be rooted in your weakest target area. All of us have weak points or systems in our bodies, the result, usually, of genetic inheritance. During the course of your life this weakness can be exacerbated by poor nutrition, overbreathing, stress, overwork, or a variety of other factors. Genetic research increasingly shows that there is such a thing as a cystic fibrosis gene, or a cancer gene. If you are born with such a gene, you will always have a vulnerability where that particular disease is concerned, although it is by no means inevitable that you will come to suffer from it. However, something such as poor nutrition could activate the program for that gene. Similarly, if your area of weakness is your circulatory system, or heart, stress or hyperventilation could cause you to suffer from a related illness. But, if you eat sensibly, exercise, manage your stress levels, and avoid hyperventilation, the danger of heart disease is dramatically diminished. The reverse is also true.

If your Control Pause is as low as 10 to 15, it is likely that you already suffer from some illness, although it may, at present, be hidden. Such conditions as diabetes, low blood pressure, tuberculosis, and even tumors can lie silent and dormant for a long time before something, perhaps a general malaise, alerts you that something is wrong. You may even have experienced some specific symptoms, without realizing what they indicated. In a few cases—that of motor neurone disease and some cancers, for example—by the time you experience symptoms and seek advice it will be too late for conventional medical help. The sad truth is that some people can have a CP as low as 15 and still feel energetic and well. It is vitally important to remember that good health goes beyond surface performance. You need to learn to listen to your body, and to pay attention to any change in normal performance or function, such as sudden headaches, recurrent breathing problems, pain of any description, or even just a general malaise. And the best measure of what is going on beneath the skin is the Control Pause technique.

Professor Buteyko says that there are almost no exceptions to the link between a person's CP and his or her general health. A person might be apparently strong, muscular, and young, but if that person's Control Pause is only 10 or 12, he or she is very ill in some way. Alarming as this truth might seem, it has to be considered.

Once again, a very low Control Pause is not cause for panic. Instead it is a welcome warning that action—immediate action—is required. The cause of your hidden hyperventilation can be reversed and we are here to show you how. You can make great strides with this book alone, but seeking guidance from a Breath Connection expert will probably hasten the reversal of your symptoms. Everyone responds better with individual help and encouragement. Dieters tend to be much more successful with group support or counseling, just as most of us feel more inspired to exercise with the help of a personal trainer, who can tailor our programs to suit our needs. Complementary medicine has always focused on the special needs of the individual, and we have seen how effective this approach can be.

With a healthy Control Pause of 50 to 60, you have perfect balanced breathing and you can relax, knowing that you are in no danger of asthma, emphysema, bronchitis, allergies, cancers, or any of the other conditions that the Breath Connection can deal with. But things can change, particularly if there is a tendency within your family to fall prey to certain types of illness, so it is wise to be watchful and have your health checked from time to time, and regularly monitor your control pause.

People with a Control Pause between 20 and 40 seconds may have already developed some of the lesser defense mechanisms against overbreathing, such as a blocked nose, susceptibility to colds and flu, snoring, and weight gain. This means you already have moderate hyperventilation and a few simple exercises will help to remedy this.

Daily technique for self-care program for healthy people

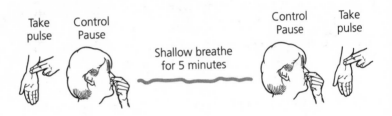

The Technique

1. As a general technique, take your pulse (see page 53) and do the Control Pause.
2. Shallow breathe for five minutes before doing another CP and then take your pulse again. Do this first thing in the morning and before going to bed.
3. Create a weekly self-care chart for yourself (see pages 243–252 for examples). It will guide you through the program and you will find it helpful to document your progress and note your improvement.

Another exercise is particularly helpful when you under stress, mentally tired, or have spent too long in front of a computer screen.

Technique to relieve a stressful situation

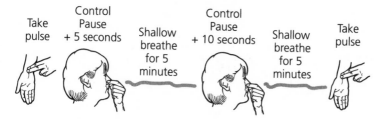

Take pulse | Control Pause + 5 seconds | Shallow breathe for 5 minutes | Control Pause + 10 seconds | Shallow breathe for 5 minutes | Take pulse

1. Take your pulse (see page 53).
2. Do the Control Pause, plus five seconds.
3. Shallow breathe for five minutes.
4. Take another CP, plus 10 seconds.
5. Shallow breathe for a further five minutes.
6. Take your pulse again.

A slightly longer exercise is recommended when you have a cold, hayfever, or flu. Do this three times a day before meals. For some people it may be advisable to reduce food intake by as much as half—but see Chapter 12. Clearly these measures would not be appropriate for an anorexic, or someone with blood sugar problems, but most people—particularly if they have a cold or flu—will benefit from eating smaller amounts without actually skipping meals. A light and simple diet puts much less strain on a network of systems already working hard to overcome a temporary disorder. Your body needs all available energy to fight illness, and you don't want to waste this precious energy on digesting a heavy meal.

1. Take your pulse.
2. Do the Control Pause.

Technique for colds, flu, and hayfever

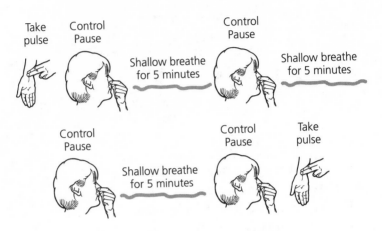

3. Shallow breathe for five minutes.

4. Another Control Pause.

5. Shallow breathe for five minutes.

6. Do another Control Pause.

7. Shallow breathe for another five minutes.

8. Do the Control Pause.

9. Take your pulse.

Before any sport, aerobics, working out in the gym, or other physical exercise, you should take your pulse, do a Control Pause, shallow breathe for five minutes, and then repeat the exercise after physical exercise and sport.

Keep your mouth closed throughout and, if necessary, find ways of reminding yourself to do so. Some people find it helpful to place little messages or even tape up posters in places where they practice the exercises, rather like those who are trying to lose weight tape pictures of obese people to

Technique for before and after physical exercise and sport

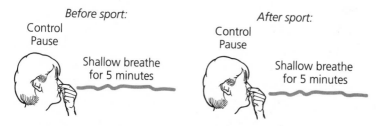

Before sport:

Control Pause

Shallow breathe for 5 minutes

After sport:

Control Pause

Shallow breathe for 5 minutes

the fridge door, or write stern little deterrents where they know they will see them.

Points to Remember

• These points apply to all of the exercises and techniques in the self-care program.

• Always keep your mouth closed at night, particularly if you snore. This will lead to a better quality of sleep. Keep it sealed with tape at work, in the car, when exercising, when you are alone, or whenever you can manage it. Affix tape vertically rather than horizontally if the latter feels too restricting.

• Put up reminder messages or stickers wherever these may be helpful. Don't feel embarrassed—tell people that you are fighting a respiratory condition, or otherwise improving your health. You may start a trend!

• Sleep in your left side (see page 52).

• Don't go to bed unless you are tired.

• Avoid dairy foods and too much protein, junk food, tea, coffee, and sugar, all of which put strain on the excretory system and can encourage the production of mucus, or encourage hyperventilation.

- Do not eat a protein meal at night
- Eat only when you are hungry, not just because it is a certain time of day (see page 189).
- Increase physical activity. While you are on the Breath Connection program, take the stairs instead of the elevator, for example, and walk to the shops instead of driving. Gardening, jogging, and even housework are all beneficial forms of exercise. Golfers should walk rather than take a golf cart.
- Almost all sport is recommended. Simply remember to check your Control Pause first and 15 minutes after you have finished and to keep your mouth closed. A lower CP after exercise indicates that you have lost too much carbon dioxide through overbreathing, so you should reduce your pace or the duration of your sporting activity until you have reconditioned your breath. Once you have learned to breathe the Breath Connection way, you will enjoy your sport or exercise much more. Swimmers, in particular, should remember to breathe through the nose only. If you want to go faster, hold your face under water long enough to take more strokes. Just don't open your mouth when you breathe.
- After driving for any distance, reading, watching TV, walking—whether on the street, field, or pitch—in fact, after any activity, get into the habit of checking your Control Pause at regular intervals so that you can see if a pattern emerges. It is helpful to see which activities cause it to rise, and which cause it to lower. It's a simple habit of self-monitoring to get into, and an instant health check.

Finally, the Breath Connection program involves the following:

- Breathing in less air than you have been used to in the past.

- Keeping your mouth closed all the time, except when eating, drinking, or talking. Tape up your mouth as often as you can and certainly when alone.

- Continuing to use steroid medication if you are using it, and retaining your preventer. Don't cease or decrease your medication until you get the OK from your Breath Connection practitioner and your own doctor.

- Avoiding overeating, oversleeping, or sleeping on your back. Get into the habit of sleeping on your left side and practice Breath Connection exercises regularly. If you are using a bronchodilator, you will reach a point where you will have no symptoms and no longer require it.

10

Breath Connection for Asthmatic Children

Any parent whose child suffers from asthma will tell you that the sight and sound of his or her small son or daughter straining to overcome an asthma attack is the most frightening and distressing experience there is.

Your child is in pain, and virtually beyond the reach of the comfort of your hands, arms, or voice, and your sense of helplessness may be compounded by sorrow if you are aware that asthma is an inherited condition. Worst of all, your child's life is in danger.

You might not suffer from asthma, but perhaps a parent or grandparent did. Many of us carry the gene that predisposes people to asthma. If you suffer from asthma, your child has a 50 percent chance of inheriting the condition. If both you and your partner are asthmatic, this figure soars to 90 percent. But inheriting the gene does not mean that your child will go on to suffer with asthma. With diet and lifestyle management, asthma can be prevented.

Not all children suffer from severe asthma. If they are lucky, they may suffer from the odd mild asthma attack, or some of the related conditions, such as eczema or hay fever. Severe asthma is quite different. Children with severe asthma may have been doomed to a lifetime of restricted physical activity, a constant fear of a sudden attack, general breath-lessness, drug dependency, social unease, and a general inability to embrace life's potential.

Professor Buteyko asserts that, whatever their genetic inheritance, all asthmatics hyperventilate. The sooner that parents can train their children not to do so, the fewer asthmatics there will be. Even if your child has severe asthma, a little concentrated work—which most children find fun—and some easy adjustments to your family lifestyle can prevent your child from enduring the many deprivations of an asthmatic life. Once your child has stopped hyperventilation and has become accustomed to a safe and sensible diet, he or she will be much safer. High stress levels, or bouts of flu, may bring occasional relapses, but breath control will enable balance to be restored quickly. Asthma is a defense mechanism against the body's loss of carbon dioxide. If there is a correct balance of oxygen and carbon dioxide in the blood, genetically weakened areas will become stronger and less susceptible to problems.

Breath Connection for Children

Many children, happily, grow out of asthma, particularly after they have learned not to hyperventilate. But this is no reason for them, or you, to endure the worries and panics that asthma can bring. If your child suffers from regular, serious asthma attacks, the constant hyperventilation may have led to more serious illness, such as diabetes, epilepsy, or cancer. The earlier you begin Breath Connection for your child, the more chance you have of preventing these conditions from developing. If your child managed to fight asthma at a relatively young age, the Breath Connection program should still be undertaken to ensure that the rest of the body is in a balanced, healthy state. Furthermore, and less seriously, training your children early will help to prevent problems such as chronic blocked noses and snoring. On a more positive note, Breath Connection will enhance your child's powers of concentration, which will help him or her to cope with stress and pressure in the future.

Is It Safe?

Parents who are concerned that their child might be troubled or traumatized by the Breath Connection program can rest assured that the vast majority of children find it great fun. Children are even more receptive than adults to the retraining methods, not surprising, perhaps, in light of the fact that their bad habits have had a shorter period of time in which to develop. Children tend to be un-self-conscious about learning techniques and treat them as a new game. The program offers parents a wonderful opportunity to create strong foundations for their child's health by training them to breathe correctly.

In the past, many doctors diagnosed any child with the slightest wheeze or touch of bronchitis as asthmatic. Drugs to treat the condition were duly prescribed. Soon, these children really did become asthmatic, as their breathing deepened, and drug intake necessarily increased. Professor Buteyko maintains that if your child is wheezy, you should not attempt to deal with the situation by giving him or her drugs. You need to train your child to breathe correctly. The wheeze itself is not dangerous—in fact, it acts as a message from the body that something might be wrong. Only when there is obvious and serious breathing difficulty should your child be given asthma medication.

Sometimes the body switches to another defense mechanism, such as eczema, one of the same family of diseases that includes asthma and a number of other allergic conditions. Some children grow out of these conditions, but it is not a good idea to wait until they do so. Professor Buteyko observed that a whole host of conditions are linked to hyperventilation, and the longer your child suffers from asthma or another problem that indicates deep, incorrect breathing, the more likely he or she is to develop one. Asthma can kill, but it can also be contained.

BARRY

On rare occasions, our advice is not enough, and we admit to feeling deep frustration and despair when this occurs. Barry was a 15-year-old with severe asthma. Before his mother brought him to us, he had been under the care of one of the country's leading respiratory specialists, but this had not prevented a frightening respiratory arrest in a hospital bathroom one night. This attack marked Barry's fourth serious crisis in four years.

Barry's mother, Sonia, had ensured that he had all the nebulizers he needed at home, in her car, and in his schoolbag, but none of these precautions comforted her much. Barry was very overweight, was bullied at school, and was unable to take part in sports or games. He was a sluggish and understandably unhappy young man. Sonia came to us without consulting Barry's existing doctors because she feared that they would be discouraging about and skeptical of Breath Connection. But Barry made extremely good progress and soon stopped needing nebulizers, taking only two or three puffs of an inhaler each day. But he simply refused to take oral steroids because he was under the impression that they were the cause of his obesity.

The irony is that he would have needed to take only two or three tablets each day, rather than the 40 or so a day that he had been given on his many emergency hospital admissions. If he had taken small doses of steroids, Barry could have coped with respiratory problems, such as a slight cough or the flu, with ease. Instead, he was hospitalized time and again for these problems, and at the hospital he was forced to take very high doses.

During one of his hospital visits, Barry told his specialist about Breath Connection. His consultant's response was to tell Barry about a wonder drug that would soon be available to deal with all of his problems. It was a drug that would have all the advantages of steroids, but no side effects. Barry was so keen to believe this, just as he had been keen to believe that he would grow out of his asthma, that he refused to take part in Breath Connection exercises from that moment onward.

He was no longer a small child, and Sonia felt unable to force him to continue. So, Barry returned to using his nebulizer four or five times a day and went back to his routine of regular hospital visits. We had not been able to convince him that small doses of correctly administered steroids would help him, and that he would, eventually, have no dependency on them as his asthma symptoms disappeared. Nor could we convince him that every aspect of his life—both now and in the future— would improve if he stuck with us.

The wonder drug on which Barry pinned his hopes never had the desired effect and he remains severely asthmatic and severely overweight—an unhappy existence for an unhappy young man. This sad story underlines how important it is to take asthmatic children to Breath Connection as soon as possible.

The Breath Connection program can significantly reduce symptoms of asthma in children and offer guidance for parents in order to help them cope. If parents are asthmatic themselves, there is even more reason to attend. Our program can train children from an early age to balance their breathing and to reduce the likelihood of developing disease in later life.

All parents want the best for their children—a good education, friends, holidays, toys, and nice clothes—but your greatest gift to your child is a foundation of good health. Without this, every aspect of a child's later life will be restricted. Elderly people may expect to have illness or disability of one form or another and, although we at Breath Connection would never advise it, it seems somehow more acceptable to allow an unhealthy state to continue. But for children who are ill, the prospect of a lifetime of ill health and disability is tragic. You as a parent can do a great deal to prevent this situation from developing, and we can show you how.

Keeping Informed

Correct information is always a good start. If, until now, your asthmatic child has been given steroids and bronchodilators, his or her symptoms may be quite minor. Don't be fooled. Your child is not free from asthma, the symptoms of the condition have merely been suppressed. The asthma exists, and its root cause, hyperventilation, must be addressed before real progress can be achieved. More asthma medication is prescribed today than it was 50 years ago, and yet the incidence of childhood asthma has soared. If your child does grow out of asthma attacks, but continues to overbreathe, his or her body will find another way of coping with the reduced levels of carbon dioxide, possibly by contracting a more serious illness. Even mild asthmatics should be encouraged to take part in a program of counterattack. The fact that your child already has asthma means that his or her health is on a slippery downward slope. Its cause is hyperventilation.

But this condition can be reversed. Your child will be able to participate fully in school life, with friends, with family, and all of the systems of his or her body will function properly. The danger of more serious illness later in life will be removed or reduced dramatically. You, in turn, will be able to relax and stop worrying about your child's future health—and you'll probably become a more relaxed and efficient parent. Whenever you are worried, you can monitor your child's progress by participating in the STEPS program (see page 149).

At the Hale Clinic, we have felt a great sense of fulfillment to see children helped by the Breath Connection program. Somehow, seeing childhood disorders corrected is one of the most exciting aspects of Breath Connection.

Children who have been diagnosed as being asthmatic should follow the subsequent program. Those with a cough and bronchitis should practice the shallow breathing exercises and a STEPS program (see page 149). We will try to make all of these activities fun, and you can do so at home as well. Charts can be filled in with colored markers or stars to record progress, and small rewards for a job well done will appeal to most children's sense of competition.

For simplicity, we have described the child as "he," but the guidelines do, obviously, apply to girls as well!

Here's how you should begin:

- Make sure your child uses his medication correctly. He should only use a bronchodilator if he his having difficulty breathing. Ensure that steroids are being taken correctly (see page 67).

- Learn as much as you can about the drugs that your child has been prescribed (see pages 59–72). If you still have questions, don't be afraid to ask your doctor to explain things further.

- Teach your child to do the Control Pause. Make it into a game.

- Stop using a peak flow meter. To assess your child's condition at any time, use the Control Pause. Listen to him when he tells you how he is feeling.

- Teach your child to keep his mouth closed when he breathes, and to keep it shut unless he is talking, eating, or drinking. Tape his mouth at night. Tape yours, too, if it helps to inspire him!

- Reduce or eliminate chocolate, cola drinks, ice cream, dairy products, and junk foods. Apart from the fact they can ruin teeth and lead to weight problems, they often have little or no nutrition and can be hard to digest. Any foods that are difficult to digest increase the body's need for carbon dioxide. Furthermore, fizzy drinks create "wind," and a further loss of carbon dioxide. Don't allow a high-protein meal within two or three hours of bedtime.

- Encourage him to sleep on his left side. If necessary, prop him up with pillows to prevent him from turning. Check that all is well several times during the night.

STEPS

STEPS should only be undertaken by children suffering from asthma or bronchitis. If, in addition to these problems, they have any of the conditions asterisked in Appendix B, they should be taken to see a Breath Connection expert rather than relying on a self-care program. A Breath Connection practitioner will be able to advise on complications and will be able to help your child to achieve excellent results. Any children with diseases other than asthma and bronchitis should be taken to see a Breath Connection expert rather than relying on a self-care program. Always check with us first, to see if we can be of assistance. There is every chance that we can help with existing illnesses, and we should certainly be able to help reduce the need for drugs. If your child suffers from a condition that involves unavoidable medication, we can provide a form of treatment to run alongside.

If your child is younger than five, it is best to attend a Breath Connection course to learn what you can do to help him. Then explain why he is doing the exercises. Try to help him to understand that taking in too much air is making him ill. It may be hard for such a young child to grasp the idea, but it is important that it is carefully explained. Never force or push a young child if he is hesitant. Instead, make it into a game, and try to ensure that he sees the exercises as a form of play. Tape the mouths of the whole family, and cut silly shapes for each family member. If the whole family is involved in the process, it is unlikely that your child will feel that he is being singled out for some kind of strange treatment.

Problems for your older child can be dealt with by following STEPS. Remember that asthma-related problems, such as a blocked nose, a cough, or shortness of breath, can cause your child to tire easily. Don't push him too far. Be gentle and patient, and the results will soon be evident.

The Technique

1. Start by taking your child's pulse. Don't worry if it seems to be a little high. Children often have higher pulses than adults.

2. Ask him to stand with his mouth closed. If his nose is blocked, ask him to breathe using a corner of his mouth only.

3. Ask him to breathe out through his nose if possible. He should hold his breath out and pinch his nose between his thumb and forefinger.

4. Ask your child to pretend that he is walking underwater, with his mouth and nose closed, and to do this for as long as he can. Count his steps and make a note of it for his chart. Encourage him as he walks.

5. As soon as your child starts to feel uncomfortable, he should begin to breathe in again shallowly. Tell him to resist the temptation to gulp when he releases his nose. Join in with him if you think it would be helpful.

6. Once he has completed his steps, he should continue to breathe shallowly with his mouth shut. Any child who began this exercise with a blocked nose will probably find that it is becoming less congested.

7. Ask your child to sit still and breathe gently—like a small mouse—for three or four minutes. To check that he is doing this correctly, put a finger under his nose to feel the airflow. It should feel very, very light. Teach your child to do this at the first sign of any asthma problem.

8. Take his pulse at the end of the STEPS program and look at his chart so that you can monitor his progress.

STEPS program for asthmatic children

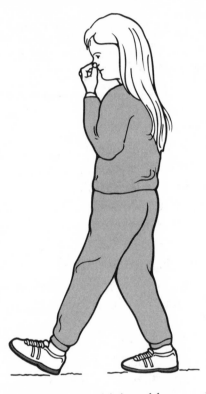

Ideally, your child should be able to take 120 steps, which is the equivalent of a Control Pause of 50 to 60 seconds. One hundred twenty steps means that he is unlikely to suffer from asthma. Don't worry unduly if he is well below that ideal 120 steps. With gentle perseverance, he can reach that figure. It is a good idea to do one daily Control Pause with your child as another way of measuring to see if his asthma is clearing or becoming worse.

Now let's imagine the day of a typical parent with a typically asthmatic child who has woken with asthma symptoms. The STEPS exercises should be performed before resorting to a bronchodilator, although this can be offered if STEPS does not work to relieve the symptoms. If it does work, congratulate your child—and yourself!

Repeat the exercise two or more times throughout the day. Quite soon, your child should be able to manage by himself if you are busy, but remind him to note or remember the number of steps he took so that these can be added to the chart. It is good for him to learn to take responsibility for his health. When your child goes to school, make sure that he has taken the required dose of steroids, if appropriate. But remind him to use his inhaler or bronchodilator only if he cannot control his symptoms with correct breathing. Ask him to keep his mouth closed whenever possible. Naturally, you will need to speak to his teachers at school to explain his problems and to enlist their support.

It is unlikely that your child will be embarrassed about his asthma. So many children suffer from it these days that at playtime children often line up for their puffers, which have been entrusted to the teacher at the start of the day. Some puffers are even designed in the shapes of animals and footballs to make them more user-friendly. We don't know whether to be heartened or discouraged by this! It all helps to reduce the stigma of asthma, but it does show that a whole industry has grown up around the manufacture of a device that should not be necessary in the first place. However, at this point in time, as many as one in four children uses a puffer or is developing asthma symptoms.

A welcome upshot of this is that few children have problems keeping their mouths closed, using tape or puffers, or otherwise following their programs in public places. Not only are there so many of them in the same boat, but they will do almost anything to be able to rush around the playground normally. Adults are far more likely to feel awkward.

After school, your child should perform the next exercise. Ask him to walk across the largest room in the house, or around the garden, if possible. His mouth should be closed. He should walk slowly at first, and then gradually increase his pace over two or three minutes. This will help him to get into the habit of walking—and, ultimately, running—with his mouth closed. Repeat the exercise two to four times, gradually increasing the time your child spends on it until he can actually run fast for 20 or 30 seconds without breathlessness. After each STEPS exercise, your child should be able to increase the time he spends walking or running, even if it is only by a few seconds. Whenever possible, stay near your child so that you can observe and note his progress.

Do the STEPS program with your child two or three times, about an hour before he goes to bed. Then tape his mouth and ensure that he falls asleep in the correct position. When you check on him during the night, replace the tape if it has been loosened. Gently close his mouth if it has fallen open.

If he has moved onto his back, slip him back onto his left side. If your child has had a history of having asthma problems at a particular time of the night, set your alarm so that you can be there with him just before that old danger point. Wake him gently if he is wheezy or if his breathing is too heavy and deep. It may sound unkind—and not much fun for you, either—but this will stop him from being violently wakened by an asthma attack. Settle your child back to sleep, cuddle him, and wait with him until he is sleeping calmly again.

The STEPS program can be adapted to fit in with whatever interest your child has. If he enjoys computer games, tell him that his asthma is an invader that has to be zapped. He could even put his daily chart onto his computer and fill it in himself on screen. A younger child could be encouraged to think of his asthma as a naughty elf who came to visit, but must now go home. Do whatever you know to be appropriate for your particular child, and do so at the earliest possible age and stage. It is important he understands that by taking part in the exercises and other aspects of the program, he is taking control of the unwelcome illness that upsets his body and stops him from doing the things he enjoys best in life.

Maintenance for Asthmatic Children

Once your child has reached 120 steps, continue practicing regularly two to three times per day for a few months. Then practice once a day for a few months and then practice once a week indefinitely.

This will enable you to monitor your child's health on a weekly basis using the STEPS program. If the number of steps starts to decrease significantly, then temporarily increase the steps program to two to three times per day until your child can reach 120 steps again.

Preventative Self-Care for Well-Being

Even if you have no reason to suppose that your child has inherited the asthma gene, and even if he suffers from no obvious respiratory illness, you will likely want to do everything in your power to encourage the kind of good health that will set him in good stead for the rest of his life. You can start by involving him in a program of preventive measures and exercise from about the age of five.

Unlike most adults, children are learning all the time—sometimes unconsciously, and sometimes with an infectious sense of wonder and enthusiasm. So take little notice if they grizzle briefly when you introduce the new routines. All children soon get used to them and usually enjoy the novelty of a new way of doing things. It is much easier to reeducate a child to breathe properly than it is to change the habits of an adult. You don't have to overstress the health angle if you feel that this aspect of the program may be a turnoff for your young Mister or Miss Cool.

Hyperventilation can affect any child at any age, and it can program a child to be vulnerable to many serious illnesses later in life. We cannot make this point too often, or too emphatically. We heartily recommend that you begin the program to protect your child's future.

The Technique

Here is the basic plan:

- Encourage him to keep his mouth closed unless speaking, eating, or drinking.
- Tape his mouth at night. As we mentioned earlier, there are now tapes with animal faces and all manner of devices that make this simple step an unthreatening game. If it's fun, your child will take part. Encourage him to sleep on the left side.
- Keep dairy foods off the table, and avoid carbonated drinks and sugar, especially early in the morning. Find deli-

cious, healthy substitutes for treats. There are many sources of calcium, other than dairy products, and you should encourage your child to eat plenty of them (see page 192).

• Encourage your child to keep his mouth closed during sports or games. If this proves difficult, try to steer him toward less strenuous outdoor activity until he is able to do so.

• Keep a close watch on all your child's breathing patterns.

• Do the Control Pause (see page 48) with him at least three or four times a day, even after he has become used to performing it by himself. It will be useful for you to observe any fluctuations, and when his levels drop, you will be alerted to take him to a Breath Connection practitioner.

• All of these measures will help your child to perform better at school, and be happier, as well as healthier. You'll be pushing at an open door as he sees for himself how much more he is enjoying every aspect of his life.

• Please note that the STEPS program is just for children with asthma or bronchitis.

Mouth Taping

A word here about the issue of mouth taping, which some parents consider to be a controversial technique. Some parents need to be persuaded to follow this advice and have to be disabused of the idea that they are being cruel to be kind. Mouth taping is not cruel. There is no pain whatsoever involved in the gentle application of a light tape. Furthermore, it is lifted off, rather than fiercely pulled, like an adhesive strip on an elbow or a grazed knee. Children tend not to be restricted by it, particularly if they have been used to wearing it at home during the day and see that their parents have also placed a strip across their own lips. Tape should always be placed vertically rather than horizontally, so that you child can easily remove it if he feels uncomfortable.

If you feel like you are imprisoning your child by using the micropore tape as he sleeps, just remember that your child can easily remove it for himself if he feels uncomfortable. Chances are that he will slip quickly into a calm and restorative sleep, and the tape will be in place the next morning. Some parents wait until their child has drifted into sleep before applying the little strip to close their mouths. That, too, is just fine.

CARL

Carl was 13 and crazy about surfing. He was determined not to let his asthma prevent him from enjoying it. He carried three Bricanol inhalers whenever he was near the waves—one strung around his neck, one in a pocket of his swimming trunks, and one taped to his surfboard. After two weeks of customized and strenuous Breath Connection exercises designed to build up his carbon dioxide levels and beat hyperventilation, Carl was able to give up all of his medication. His father, a businessman, gave a lunch party for all of the members of his staff who wanted to learn more about the balanced breathing techniques that had saved his son.

The Severely Asthmatic Child

Severely asthmatic children will have had to be hospitalized at least once because of their asthma. Undoubtedly, you were frightened by any attack that led to hospitalization and are determined that such an attack will never occur again. This is what you must do.

First of all, ask yourself why it happened. Think carefully. Was it hyperventilation? A lack of steroids, particularly as your child's condition became critical? Almost certainly your child was given massive doses of bronchodilator drugs (nebulizers) and put on oxygen for some time after his admission. When you were with him, did you have the correct information and the right drugs on hand so that you could insist that the dosage was correct for him?

No one wants to be pessimistic, but if an emergency does occur, we do feel that you should be there to inform his carers about his previous conditions and actually insist that you have a small dose of oral steroids ready for him to take when the need arises. You need to be in charge and should not have to wait for well-meaning, but possibly misinformed, doctors to decide your child's fate. Doctors normally respect the health records that diabetics carry with them, and the same should apply to asthmatics. A smaller dose of steroids, regularly administered, is likely to be much more effective than huge, emergency doses for any asthmatic—adult or child.

Here is an example of the same type of concept. Sunlight can, in moderation, be very beneficial. Too much of it, too quickly, can be extremely harmful. Steroids are much the same. A little, moderate dose is fine. Too much, and it puts enormous strain on the system.

Be firm and insist on supervising the drugs that your child is given during an emergency, and the rate at which the dosage is administered. Oral steroids should only be necessary if a single puff of Ventolin does not bring relief. One tablet, chewed, with a drink of warm water, should help. Don't allow another one to be administered for an hour or two. Then keep going until the child is clearly more comfortable. Don't worry too much about oxygen. The air around you has enough, and he will not need to be given any more. Later, ensure that your child only takes steroids when there is obvious distress. Seeing that his breathing is regulated is the main thing, so don't let yourself be bamboozled into agreeing to large doses of unnecessary drugs.

When your child is safely back at home, try to keep to your normal routine. Stick to his exercises, and make sure that his diet is sensible. Don't push him to eat if he has no appetite, and don't be tempted to put rewards such as chocolate bars in his school lunchbox. You are likely to feel so relieved he is on the mend that you will give into any demand, but be firm! Apples, bananas, honey, cereal bars, and other such things can be just as delicious.

When he is ready to begin school, continue with your discipline and remind him to stick to the "mouth-closed" routines. This shouldn't be a contentious request, since the very recent memory of his crisis will still be fresh in his mind and he will want to do anything to avoid that trauma again. Quietly tell his teachers about the attack so that they can be particularly observant. Remind them that however plaintive he might be, he should not be allowed to participate in sports or organized games quite yet. He may also need his teacher's encouragement and reminders to keep his mouth shut. He should be allowed to keep his puffer in his pocket at this time, rather than hand it over to a teacher. You will have told him when and how to use it.

Remind your child to take his bronchodilator when he needs it—not when anyone else tells him to. Ensure that he has one or two tablets of oral steroids in his bag, and remind him how and when to use them.

After school, collect your child in the usual way and make sure that you behave as if things were quite normal again. Subtly, however, you should encourage him to continue with his breathing exercises, and not feed him until he is hungry. Without making a great deal of fuss, you must spend extra time with him, especially before he goes to bed at night, to note his changing condition. Open the window as he gets sleepy, and make sure that his mouth is taped and that he is in the right position for restful sleep. Check on him up to five times during the night while he is still in recovery from a severe attack.

Refuse any offers of antiflu vaccines or any other conventional safeguards for the time being. You are doing well enough, and he does not need a vaccine that might weaken his immune system and trigger a further attack. Dismiss any offers of techniques that are based upon increasing the lung capacity of your child or methods that claim to clear mucus. By now, you know that mucus is a friendly defense mechanism.

We are in the process of converting your child's severe asthma to mild asthma. You've been through and weathered a crisis. You are on course, and it's important that you don't let anyone misdirect you.

Summary for All Parents

- Introduce the Breath Connection program as a game, which will help your child to take control of his condition.
- Where appropriate, do the STEPS exercise three times a day with your child, especially before bed.
- Ensure that your child's mouth is closed when he sleeps. Use micropore tape (see page 51), if necessary.

See that he sleeps correctly, propped up on his left-hand side.

- Avoid giving foods that we have warned against (see page 191).
- Follow the self-care program so that your child can learn the best habits in the best possible environment—the family home.
- Congratulate yourself—you are doing wonderful work!

11

Breath of Life

By now you are aware of the dangers of taking in too much air, or hyperventilating. In this chapter, we go a little deeper into the thinking behind this central, essential principle. We explain in more detail why unbalanced breathing can be so harmful and why it sets the stage for a whole host of health problems.

In some circumstances, Professor Buteyko was able to offer a clear explanation of how overbreathing damages specific bodily functions and systems, why it becomes the vehicle or channel for certain disorders. In other cases, the professor noted an empirical link between hyperventilation and illness, in that when a patient's breathing became balanced, the disease disappeared even though there was no precise physiological explanation for this.

The idea that carbon dioxide is at best a waste gas and at worst a poisonous one has become so fixed that until now minimal research into its uses and importance has taken place. One of our great hopes is that this book will inspire further research into the role that this natural gas can play in alleviating a huge range of disorders. Some readers may still wonder how something as simple and automatic as breathing could possibly be at the root of so many illnesses. While it is fairly obvious how incorrect breathing can affect respiratory disorders, you may find it hard to see how carbon dioxide deprivation can account for a raft of other conditions, ranging from angina to varicose veins.

Think of it in this way: Our planet's atmosphere is made up of many gases, primarily carbon dioxide and oxygen. Changes in the balance of these gases over the centuries have led to huge environmental disruption. Humans have also evolved and developed over the centuries, and not always at the same pace as the radical environmental changes. Shifts in the balance of these important gases in the environment affect us all. It is a great pity that more medical research has not been devoted to addressing the importance of the way we breathe and the relationship between the two key gases that we require to do so. There has been a huge lack of research into the way that our body systems respond to these gases and how our changing environment may have affected our overall health. Breathing, oxygen, and carbon dioxide hold the answers to many of the illnesses that have baffled doctors and scientists for many years.

Those of you who already suffer from asthma, emphysema, bronchitis, or any of the other disorders listed in Appendix B may only be interested in dealing with your diagnosed disease. But the Breath Connection program can also help you to avoid falling prey to new illnesses and can help you to avoid a huge range of nonrespiratory illnesses. We cannot stress too strongly how a deprivation of carbon dioxide influences many, many body functions, as well as our body's performance and its ability to react to hostile circumstances.

Although every physiology is unique, we can confidently make some generalizations that apply to everyone.

There is a common, modern belief that our capacity for good or poor health is genetically predicated and that there is little we can do to change our destiny. At Breath Connection, we believe that every individual has the power to overcome a huge number of genetic disadvantages, if and when he or she needs to. Many of our weak, genetically inherited areas can be identified by a cool review of lifestyle and may be positively changed where necessary. We can't change the color of our eyes, gender, basic shape, hair color, personality, or IQ— at least not without varying degrees of effort and artifice. But in many cases, we can improve our health naturally and, in some cases, with very little effort.

Our Genetic Legacy

Our genes have bestowed one legacy, but, with the benefit of modern science, we have, today, more flexibility than ever before. We now have the wherewithal to counter many of the inherited factors that we cannot live with. Many of us can reduce the risks that genetics play with our health, regardless of our priorities. Whether you want to live longer, or better, or whether you want to slow down the physical signs of aging, help is at hand. This book isn't about beauty or cosmetic issues, but we do appreciate that this may be a factor for some readers. The Breath Connection program improves health on all levels and makes a very noticeable improvement in the way you look and feel.

There is little that we can do about the environment that we live in; all of us can play a small part in helping to green our lifestyles, but we are, in the end, stuck with existing pollution, food additives, and other factors that influence our health. There are, however, many things that we can do, on an individual basis, to minimize the effects of our environment. Lifestyle changes can reduce the overall burden on the body and make it easier for our bodies to cope with the demands placed upon it.

As an individual, you can stop smoking, reduce your alcohol consumption, especially spirits, and cut down on red meat and other proteins. Seek quality rather than quantity when you are choosing foods, and avoid those that have been processed and altered with additives and other modifications. Get more regular exercise. This advice is basic for anyone who has ever taken steps to improve health, but it cannot be stressed too often. What may not be clear is the fact that you can strengthen any genetic weaknesses by creating a lifestyle that is conducive to good health. And, even better, you can strengthen your body even further by reconditioning your breathing.

As you know, illness of many kinds is often the result of a carbon dioxide deficiency. In this chapter, we look at the way that this deprivation can affect a series of essential bodily functions, including the cardiovascular, digestive, eliminatory, hormonal, and immune systems, as well as brain and respiratory function. We show how the efficiency of each of these systems relies not merely upon balanced breathing, but upon complete and harmonious interaction between all the systems. This is the basis of holistic treatment, for whole health.

A Holistic Approach

Many of our doctors hold the view that illness needs only to be treated when it occurs. When illness strikes, the affected part or system is treated, but the rest of the body, including emotional factors, is generally ignored. We believe that illness is part of an overall process and the result of an imbalance within the body itself. There is no point in treating only one part, when the cause is an overall imbalance. Taking the example of a car manufacturer once again, doctors are happy to change tires, replace spark plugs, or tune a faulty engine, but they aren't happy to recommend a complete engine check or a broadscale service. We believe that all of the parts work in tandem and are inextricably linked. The health of one system undoubtedly affects the health of every other system in the body. Once again, this is the basis of holistic medicine. Breath Connection offers holistic treatment. It aims to provide an optimum level of carbon dioxide so that all your vital organs and systems are oxygenated and all-around health is achieved.

As we look at each of the physiological systems in turn, try to think of them as interconnecting cogs. When they are all running smoothly, your body functions well. A blockage or something out of sync in any of these cogs can affect all of the other cogs and trigger disease, usually in the area in which you are genetically predisposed to be weak.

Conditions ranging from angina to epilepsy are caused by hyperventilation. What we call *disease* can often simply be a manifestation of carbon dioxide deprivation.

In each section, we explain the role that carbon dioxide plays and what illnesses could manifest in your body when you have a weakness in that area. We also give you an idea of what to expect when things have been righted. Never forget that your own will has a major part to play in all this and participating in the Breath Connection program is part of your choice to take control of a longer and more fulfilling life. As a bonus, reconditioning your breathing may well enhance the quality of the genes you pass on to future generations. We know that if we damage our cellular structure and produce dysfunctional genetic changes through, for example, what we eat (many food additives have been found to be mutative, tending to affect the genetic pattern that is passed on to unborn children), we can be creating genetic problems in our children and our children's children. By improving the quality of what we eat and drink, by ensuring that our bodies are working at optimum levels, by aiming for a balanced mental condition, and by eschewing smoking, drinking, recreational drugs, and too much ultraviolet light, we are safeguarding our genetic template not just for ourselves but for our present and future families.

Even if you do not suffer from illness in any of the specific areas we cover, remember that hyperventilation creates an environment within the body for disease to take hold. Although you may be experiencing good health at present, the stage will have been set for illness, in whichever part of the body you have a weakness. Breath Connection is preventative medicine; you can reduce your chances of suffering from illness at a later date by creating a healthy body environment now.

As you learn to recondition your breathing, you will notice an improvement in many bodily functions. Your metabolism will probably speed up so that you will absorb nutrients such as vitamins and minerals more rapidly, and, although you will have more energy, you will be inclined to eat less if you are overweight. Anorexics will recover some of their appetite. Most allergies will disappear as you create the correct acid-alkaline (pH) balance, and your elimination system will improve dramatically. In fact, a major detoxification of the body will begin and you will become less vulnerable to the minor infections and diseases that are environmental hazards for us all.

The test of any theory is "does it work in practice?" Many people in the United Kingdom and in Australia have already enjoyed huge benefits from taking part in the Breath Connection program, particularly with respiratory conditions such as asthma, emphysema, and bronchitis. Many others conditions, listed in Appendix B, have been relieved significantly.

Learning to recondition the breathing is a major part of preventative health care, as important as nutrition and exercise. This system represents nothing less than the birth of a new medical system, which heralds one of the most exciting, important, and far-reaching medical breakthroughs of the century.

Respiration

ASSOCIATED DYSFUNCTIONAL CONDITIONS:

ASTHMA, EMPHYSEMA, BRONCHITIS, BREATHLESSNESS, CHRONIC FATIGUE, SNORING, INSOMNIA, SLEEP APNEA, CYSTIC FIBROSIS, BLOCKED NOSE, SINUSITIS

We have learned that respiratory illness is not caused by getting too little air, but by inhaling too much. In fact, some sufferers inhale as much as eight times more than the healthy norm. Hyperventilation reduces the carbon dioxide stored in the alveoli of the lungs, and one way the body copes with this is to close down the airways. The tragedy of taking drugs such as those contained in bronchodilators is that they unnaturally dilate the bronchial tubes to facilitate breathing, yet dilated air passages are the cause of the attack in the first place. Not only are such manufactured drugs addressing only symptoms and responses, but they fail to deal with the cause of the problem and actually make it much, much worse. While drugs may offer brief relief in the short term, in the long term, they suppress symptoms and aggravate the condition.

Carbon dioxide is nature's own bronchodilator. When the level of carbon dioxide in the lungs is maintained, the body does not need to go into spasm to reduce the intake of breath. One exercise for children (see pages 150–155) instantly boosts the level of carbon dioxide in the body and can be used instead of drugs to give instant relief from the spasms, wheezing, dizziness, and coughing associated with respiratory disorders. More important, by completely reconditioning the breathing, the original problems can be circumvented and fewer, if any, attacks will be experienced in the future.

Take Care

Almost 4 million people in the United Kingdom suffer from asthma, and about a third of those cases are serious. We know that the condition kills about 2,000 people every year, a figure that triples in the United States. Despite being linked with atmospheric pollution and other external factors (such as allergens, pollen, house dust, animal hair, mold, fungi spores, climate, temperature, and stress), asthma was comparatively rare even 75 years ago, when parts of the world were arguably more polluted.

Asthma has been recognized by physicians for hundreds of years, and it has not been considered to be a serious illness until the 1930s. While no statistics on the death rate of asthmatics in the distant past are available, we can certainly see a general trend emerging in the twentieth century. As the century nears its end, it is clear, beyond all doubt, that asthma is a very significant cause of premature death. It's time we took it more seriously. Here's a brief history of our approach to asthmatic disease:

• In 1794, the distinguished Edinburgh physician Cullen wrote: "The asthma, though often threatening immediate death, seldom occasions it, and many persons have lived long under this disease." Sir William Osler wrote: "Death during the attack is unknown." (Young J. Pentland, 1892)

• A nineteenth-century dictionary of medicine includes the following entry: "Patients rarely, if ever, die of spasmodic asthma. Though death may ensue from some of its complications and sequels, and the disease being a functional one, cannot be said to have any morbid anatomy."

• J.J. Conybeare's 1929 textbook (Livingstone) states: "It is doubtful whether death has ever been caused by uncomplicated asthma [asthma without emphysema]. Nor does asthma tend necessarily to shorten life. Asthma is compatible with long life, and many chronic asthmatic patients live to a good old age and die of some other ailment at the last."

• In his 1930 volume, *The Treatment of Asthma* (M.K. Lewis), Dr. A. H. Douthwaite wrote: "The prognosis of bronchial asthma is one of the greatest difficulty. So far as longevity is concerned, the outlook is not necessarily adversely affected. Many asthmatics live well past middle age, for they seem to be less prone to other diseases which are apt to rise in the fifth decade. Family longevity is a point to be borne in regard to the future."

• Dr. W. Fox, a general practitioner since 1931, and author of the book *Asthma* (Robert Hale, 1995), was one of the first doctors to raise the alarm. He said: "What is going on here? Here we are, in 1992, in the grip of a worldwide epidemic of asthma deaths and only a few years ago our clinical ancestors were calmly saying that it never happened. Were they all blind? It seems hardly likely since death from asthma suffocation is a particularly horrifying spectacle, and the medical giants of the past were so impressed by the curious benignity of asthma that they all mentioned it."

• In an uncanny representation of Professor Buteyko's own thinking, Dr. Fox continued: "The physicians' approach —if effective—must inevitably cause deaths, and the apparent harmlessness of asthma up to the recent past is because the medicines used in those days were ineffective."

• Opinions down the ages seem to support our view that asthma need not be a killer. Yet Dr. Douthwaite was writing at a time when Britain's cities were frequently cloaked in filthy industrial smog and many, if not most, of today's wonder drugs had yet to be developed. Ironically, the dramatic increase in asthma in the Western world—to near epidemic levels—comes at a time when the amount of asthma medications being prescribed is at an all-time high. We have to ask the question: Why, today, with the millions being spent on asthma research both in the United Kingdom and United States, is asthma getting worse, not better?

• In 1997, Dr. Richard Norton observed in *Wheeze of the World* that while Ethiopian peasants don't get asthma, wealthy Europeans do. Prior to unification, asthma was far more prevalent in West Germany than in East Germany, despite the fact that the East had much greater pollution problems and its inhabitants had severely limited access to medication. This paradox remains: The more we learn about it, the less able we, in the West, seem to be able to control asthma. Researchers come up with many theories about asthma's causes and subdivide these into reasons behind different types of asthma—allergic, nonallergic, emotional, environmental, and so on. They have, however, sought in vain to identify the actual root cause.

Overbreathing

Breathing through your mouth, as many people with respiratory disorders habitually do, involves inhaling larger quantities of air than is necessary. Apart from detrimentally affecting your carbon dioxide levels and increasing the risk of breathing in allergens, mouth-inhaled air can irritate the airways, resulting in inflammation, constriction, and excessive mucus production, often leading to a blocked nose and sinusitis. When the airways are narrowed, breathing becomes labored. This can lead to a panic attack, which causes you to gasp for air and compound the situation. Furthermore, the low carbon dioxide levels found in asthmatics reduce the body's ability to produce the natural form of the hormone cortisone and this can leave the body vulnerable to allergic responses.

Chronic Fatigue Syndrome (CFS)

Another disease of the respiratory system is chronic fatigue, but sufferers are seldom aware that they are overbreathing. Due to the Verigo/Bohr effect (see page 240), sufferers feel tired when their muscles do not receive enough oxygen. Fit people will feel healthily tired after exercise because they have used up oxygen stored in the muscles, but this is quickly replenished with rest. If you have chronic fatigue syndrome, your muscles are losing oxygen because of incorrect breathing, not through physical exertion. Hyperventilation can also prevent blood flow to the brain, leading to dizziness and loss of concentration and memory. Other symptoms include weakness, exhaustion, sleep disturbance, breathlessness, heartburn, cramps, and pins and needles.

Chronic fatigue syndrome

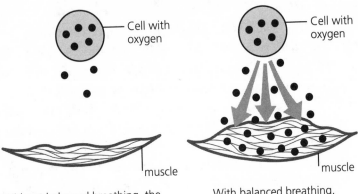

Without balanced breathing, the oxygen in the cell is not released into the muscle, causing the muscle tiredness of chronic fatigue.

With balanced breathing, the oxygen in the cell is released into the muscle.

The diagram shows how oxygen feeds the muscles. With CFS, the oxygen becomes tied to the hemoglobin due to the Verigo/Bohr effect (see page 240) and is not released into the cells. The large circle containing smaller ones shows how oxygen is unable to reach the muscles.

Sleep Disorders

Snoring, insomnia, and loss of breath during sleep are also symptomatic of malfunction in the respiratory center of the brain and are caused by hyperventilation. We know that snorers are more likely to develop high blood pressure and heart problems than nonsnorers and snoring can be the first stage of sleep apnea, a condition in which episodes of temporary cessation of breathing, lasting 10 seconds or longer, occur during sleep. This condition requires you to sleep with a special machine in your bedroom and kills more people than asthma does. It is vital that all snorers tape up their mouths, sleep on their left sides, and follow the Breath Connection program, first, to stop their snoring but also to prevent the later development of much more serious conditions.

GORDON

Gordon was 43, married, and a senior executive in a multinational computer company. He suffered from one of the most terrifying of the respiratory conditions—sleep apnea. In this condition, people unaccountably stop breathing while asleep. If they don't wake, they will die. Many sufferers are so frightened by the consequences of this condition that they are unable to sleep at night and get by with short naps throughout the day.

Gordon was becoming something of a social embarrassment, falling asleep at social events and even at the dinner table. His snoring had already caused his wife to sleep in another room and being alone at night had probably increased his fear of suffering an attack of sleep apnea. He was puffy and overweight and had more or less given up on his condition, after years of quick-fix diets. He had slept with a sleep apnea rescue machine in his room for two years, but when he gave up on this too, his daytime lapses into sleep became much worse.

Gordon had a very low Control Pause when he first came to Breath Connection. During his first week he learned how to breathe with a closed mouth. After a few days he had learned how to sleep comfortably for a few hours each night, without his machine, and this soon increased to half the night. Five weeks after beginning the course, Gordon could sleep through the night without his machine and his sleep apnea had begun to improve. His weight began to decrease, and he lost about 14 pounds during the first week of the course. After three months, he had shed nearly 55 pounds.

His Control Pause rose to 24, and, feeling rested, slimmer, and altogether better, he set about improving his health even further.

To summarize, it has been estimated that only 10 percent of the population naturally breathe in the correct way. Breathing correctly means breathing slowly and shallowly. As with any habit, particularly one acquired over a lifetime, training yourself to breathe differently may feel awkward at first. The breath reduction exercises you will learn during the five-day Breath Connection program will introduce you to a new way of breathing that will not only reduce any existing respiratory problems but have a hugely beneficial effect on other areas of your body.

In neither Papua New Guinea nor Ethiopia do people deep breathe. They have, moreover, no word for asthma. We in the "civilized" West have been inured with the idea that deep breathing is both natural and healthy despite the fact that there has never been any scientific evidence to suggest this is the case. Professor Buteyko sees asthma as a disease of so-called civilization.

Cardiovascular Conditions

ASSOCIATED DYSFUNCTIONAL CONDITIONS:
ANGINA, HEART FAILURE, PALPITATIONS, HIGH AND LOW BLOOD PRESSURE, MIGRAINE, IMPOTENCE

Shortage of carbon dioxide constricts the cardiovascular vessels. Although it is not as visibly obvious as it is with respiratory diseases, a shortage of carbon dioxide reduces circulation in the arterial vessels (the heart, brain, liver, and kidneys) and expands the vein vessels. Depending on where your weakest areas are, this can result in conditions such as a blocked nose, hemorrhoids, or varicose veins as well as more serious threats to health. It can lead to problems with circulation, which in itself is responsible for a whole host of other conditions. When the blood circulation malfunctions due to a need for more carbon dioxide, a strong spasm of the brain vessels can occur, particularly if other factors such as loud noises, particular foods, and a lack of sleep are involved. For some people the result is a migraine headache.

The Hyperventilation Syndrome

In common with those who researched Viagra, we at Breath Connection regard impotence as a vascular problem. By breathing correctly, the blood circulation to the penis is improved, thereby sustaining and lengthening the duration of erection. Often, patients with diabetes, heart problems, and blood pressure also suffer from impotence. All of these conditions are linked to hyperventilation.

Angina is another example of an illness affected by this malfunction of blood vessels due to carbon dioxide deficiency, as are heart palpitations. According to Professor Buteyko, most heart surgery could be avoided if patients were trained not to overbreathe. Moreover, if someone has already had a heart operation, learning to breathe the right way can prevent new heart problems from occurring.

High blood pressure is also linked to a carbon dioxide deficiency in the cardiovascular system. Overbreathing constricts or narrows the brain vessels, as Professor Gavin Andrews of St. Vincent's Hospital in Australia confirms:

> The body has to increase the blood pressure to secure normal oxygenation of the brain. Your doctor then measures your blood pressure and prescribes tablets for high blood pressure for the rest of your life. Ironically the body wants to keep your blood pressure high in order to get oxygen to the brain yet these pills will lower your blood pressure and do the opposite of what your body really needs. However, unless the condition is recognized as being caused by hyperventilation/overbreathing, it is necessary to take such pills in order to prevent a stroke or heart attack. Such medication may make a person look healthy by lowering their blood pressure, but they are not really healthy because the root cause has not been addressed. By retraining the breathing the blood pressure will return to normal and proper oxygenation of the brain will re-occur so the medication can be reduced in consultation with your doctor.

According to statistics, low blood pressure causes more heart attacks and strokes than high blood pressure and is another symptom of overbreathing. When following the Breath Connection program, all blood pressure or heart conditions must be supervised by an experienced and qualified Breath Connection practitioner.

The program can actually help to prevent strokes. People who have suffered a stroke in the past will often breathe with their mouths open, a sign of hyperventilation. And during a stroke, the person suffers from lack of oxygen to the brain. Subsequent Breath Connection exercises bring that oxygen back to the parts of the brain not permanently damaged by the stroke, so that in many cases the patient is able to regain mobility and speech.

The Digestive System

ASSOCIATED DYSFUNCTIONAL CONDITIONS:

IRRITABLE BOWEL SYNDROME, CONSTIPATION, FLATULENCE, BLOATING OF THE STOMACH, BELCHING, HEARTBURN, ULCERS, ACIDOSIS ALKALOSIS

When carbon dioxide is dissolved in water (of which our bodies comprise over 70 percent), it is converted into carbonic acid. This splits into bicarbonate ions and hydrogen ions and affects the delicate acid-alkali (pH) balance of the blood. This balance profoundly affects every chemical reaction and process in the body. All areas of the body have distinct pH levels that need to be controlled. These levels range from the extremely acidic (pH = 2) fluids in the stomach to the alkaline juices (pH = 7.5 to 8.8) in the pancreas. The pH of the blood is slightly alkaline and even a very slight shift in its balance can have dire consequences. No one can live more than a few hours if this balance shifts significantly.

Bicarbonates formed from dissolved carbon dioxide act as buffers within the body and help to neutralize acids and maintain the body's optimally alkaline state, which is very important for digestion. A balanced pH level in the blood is maintained through respiration. It is particularly affected by carbon dioxide levels. Hyperventilation causes us to breathe out more carbon dioxide than we should and is responsible for a corresponding shift in the blood's pH value to a more allergic state. Oxygen is alkaline and carbon dioxide is acidic. The essential balance between these two is needed for the digestive system to work properly. A low level of carbon dioxide in the lungs leads to respirator alkalosis, meaning an excess of alkaline reserves in the blood. This makes the body much more susceptible to viruses, allergies, cramps, and convulsions and explains why people with this area of weakness are more prone to colds and flu than others are. No one is quite sure why, but it is thought that this alkaline blood leads to inflammation and swelling of the lung lining.

It also results in spasms within the bronchial tubes and an imbalance of the metabolic processes—leading to the condition that we call asthma. A drop in the blood's carbon dioxide content of just 3 percent can upset the pH balance to such a level that death is the result. The link between respiration and health is critical, and carbon dioxide plays a crucial role in the balance.

Once the pH of your body is upset, your entire immune system is affected. A weakened immune system allows adverse conditions, such as colds and cancer, to thrive. We cannot claim to cure cancer, but following the Breath Connection program can often lead to a substantial extension of life span and improve the quality of life as well. Even in the terminal stages of cancer, the program offers pain relief without resort to such drugs as morphine. This leads to a more peaceful passing.

The Excretory (Elimination) System

ASSOCIATED DYSFUNCTIONAL CONDITIONS:
CONSTIPATION, DIARRHEA, FLATULENCE, BLOATING OF THE STOMACH

Our human waste-disposal and detoxification systems are especially important today, when our bodies are likely to be assaulted by chemicals and pesticides in the food chain and water supply however carefully we try to avoid them. This century, we have been introduced to 70,000 new chemicals in the environment. Much of our food is processed, especially junk food, and the poisons it creates need to be eliminated properly. You have only to look at a friend (or yourself) after a monitored fast or a stay at a health farm where a detoxification program has been followed to see the difference. Bloating has disappeared and weight has been reduced. The skin will have a healthier glow and there will be much more visible as well as invisible energy. A detox can be a vital part of treatments for a range of conditions from common colds to serious cancers.

However, when we hyperventilate we prevent our liver and kidneys—the organs responsible for flushing out toxic waste—from functioning properly. Lack of carbon dioxide, leading to unbalanced pH, makes it very difficult for cells in these purification machines to regenerate. Apart from contributing to many disorders of the nervous system and to the development of some cancers, this leads also to premature aging of the body.

The Breath Connection program has a major detoxing affect and greatly speeds up the elimination process. Many people with asthma who embark on the program find that they have diarrhea initially or that their feces loosen up considerably during the first days of the course. This is perfectly natural. Often our feces are not properly eliminated and stick to the walls of the colon, slowly spreading toxins throughout the body. This can lead to gastrointestinal and autoimmunity disorders including celiac disease, ulcerative colitis, Crohn's disease, and headaches. By balancing your breathing, the unwanted substances that trigger such problems are effectively flushed out of the body.

Where serious poisoning derives from external factors such as the tragic and dramatic fallout from the radiation spill at Chernobyl and the chemical warfare conducted during the Gulf War, the Breath Connection program can also assist recovery. Professor Buteyko's methods have been used in Chernobyl and received official recognition for results from the Russian government. We believe that similar results could be achieved with Gulf War Syndrome patients.

The former Soviet Union's Institute for Cosmic Medicine also embraced new ideas that have been proven to work. It focuses on the best medical care for its astronauts and Professor Buteyko's breathing methods are taught for application during space travel.

The Nervous System

ASSOCIATED DYSFUNCTIONAL CONDITIONS:
DIZZINESS, LACK OF COORDINATION, INSOMNIA, STRESS, IRRITABILITY, ALLERGIES, EPILEPSY

Carbon dioxide is used to tranquilize humans and animals. Air containing 10 percent CO_2 would make you feel distinctly dizzy. If that level was doubled, you would probably lose consciousness. At more than 20 percent, you might die. Your body is extremely sensitive to changes in the level of carbon dioxide that it inhales—much less so with oxygen. On average, each breath that you take contains about 20 percent oxygen, but even if that were to be increased by 400 percent, you probably wouldn't notice it. Only when the level dropped to below 15 percent in high altitudes would you experience distress.

As your body is 50 times more sensitive to carbon dioxide than it is to oxygen it is important that you learn about the effects that it has on all the essential systems. A decreased level of just 0.1 percent can cause dizziness, palpitations, wheezing, and a blocked nose—in short, an asthma attack. A similar increase would reverse the process.

Carbon dioxide, therefore, helps to regulate the nervous system's activity. This is why people in primitive cultures have practiced overbreathing for centuries in order to produce the heightened excitement required during certain rituals and states of altered consciousness. As an occasional activity, this probably does no long-term harm, but habitual overbreathing results in the malfunctions previously noted.

When considering the nervous system—that which affects the brain, spinal cord, peripheral nerves, and sensory organs— it is worth considering the words written by consultant chest physician L. Lum in the *Chest, Heart and Stroke Journal* (Chest, Heart, and Stroke Association): "Carbon dioxide is not just a waste gas. It plays an important function in governing bodily functions." In his book, *Epilepsy* (Oxford University Press, 1981), Anthony Hopkins states that hyperventilation is frequently used as a test procedure in treating epilepsy by inducing an epileptic fit through deliberately overbreathing. Hopkins also remarks that hyperventilation is a "trade name" for stress.

Neurological Function
- Is the principal regulator of the internal pH balance of the sensory and motor neurons of the brain
- Influences the transmission of nervous impulses at the

synapses (the junction between the neurons or their contact with a muscle cell or gland cell)

- Affects the amount of activity in the automatic nervous system and thus controls the state of balance between sympathetic and hostile activity—our "flight or fight" responses

The Hormonal (Endocrine) System

ASSOCIATED DYSFUNCTIONAL CONDITIONS:
PREMENSTRUAL SYNDROME (INCLUDING TENSION), ALLERGIES, INFERTILITY, AND MENOPAUSAL, THYROID, AND GYNECOLOGICAL PROBLEMS

Hormones are special chemicals that are secreted through the bloodstream by the endocrine glands. These include the pituitary gland, which regulates our growth, and the thyroid, which, as well as regulating our metabolic rates, governs the testes and ovaries that produce our sex hormones. Professor Buteyko found that balancing the breath was good for infertility and contributed to treatment of menstrual, pregnancy, menopausal, postmenopausal, and postnatal problems.

SARAH AND JANINE

Sarah attended a Breath Connection course because of severe and frequent migraines. She did not even mention to her practitioner that she was having trouble conceiving. Within three weeks of starting to balance her breath she found that she was pregnant, after eight years of trying.

Similarly, Janine had been drawn to Breath Connection because of panic attacks. She was so badly affected by traffic that she kept her eyes tightly shut as her husband drove her to the clinic. In social situations, she would freeze, and she often felt like crying in public. This forced her to give up her job. Even simple activities such as shopping and pleasurable ones such as outings to the theater or eating in restaurants were ordeals for Janine. Like Sarah, she did not mention her infertility problem when she came to see us. When she found that she was pregnant, just weeks into her regime, she had the added happy bonus of finding she was able to go shopping for all the things she would need for the baby.

Just a small secretion of natural chemicals from the endocrine glands can produce a dramatic response in the target cells with which they are compatible. As with all other systems in the body, hormonal activity is part of a balanced and interdependent control system. When we consider the link between the hormonal system and carbon dioxide, we should bear in mind what Yale University's Professor Y. Henderson had to say: "Carbon dioxide is the chief hormone of the entire body; it is the only one that is produced by every tissue and that probably acts on every organ."

Through the effects of increased CO_2 on the hormonal system, the pancreas functions more efficiently, therefore the metabolism speeds up, food is absorbed much better and the appetite is considerably reduced, leading to weight loss in overweight and obese people as their food cravings diminish. As we noted earlier, the Breath Connection program has the miraculous effect of stimulating appetite in anorexics as their balance is restored by correct breathing.

The Immune System

ASSOCIATED DYSFUNCTIONAL CONDITIONS:
ALLERGIES, AIDS, CHRONIC FATIGUE SYNDROME (CFS), SKIN DISEASES

The body is incredibly well designed and under normal circumstances can efficiently rally its own defenses against infections, viruses, and other invaders. However, our immune system can be severely challenged if we are breathing incorrectly and, as we learned from looking at the digestive system, when the body's pH balance is upset and the immune system is weakened, it becomes harder for the body to fight off disease. A weakened body is also more susceptible to allergies, among other things.

Many allergy tests show that many people have a sensitivity to a wide range of foods and substances, including wheat, dairy foods, chocolate, and fruit, as well as grass, pollens, and even fabric softeners. But, although these triggers may cause symptoms, they are not, in fact, the cause of the allergy. An allergy exists when the immune system is weakened. We believe that a weakened immune system is a result of hyperventilation.

When your immune system is working under par, it creates a fertile ground for allergies to develop. This explains why people with strong immune activity are able to eat and drink common allergens without any problems. It also explains why even healthy, typically nonallergic people can experience reactions to foods and substances when they are run-down—following a bout of flu, for example.

Immunity is a subject that is gathering huge scientific

attention of late, and there are many theories regarding its function and dysfunction. For example, HIV and AIDS have continued to flummox the medical profession, as has chronic fatigue syndrome and ME. What we do know, however, is that AIDS sufferers and people who are HIV positive have immune systems that have been seriously damaged.

For anyone who suffers from an immune-related condition, well-being can be vastly improved by following the Breath Connection program in conjunction with other treatments.

Brain Function

ASSOCIATED DYSFUNCTIONAL CONDITIONS:
ANXIETY, PANIC ATTACKS, INSOMNIA, DIZZINESS, MEMORY LOSS, CONCENTRATION PROBLEMS, DEPRESSION, STRESS

Carbon dioxide controls the flow of blood to the brain. When there is a low level of carbon dioxide in the blood—a condition called *hypocarbia*—blood flow is reduced, causing constriction of the blood vessels. This can lead to a whole range of conditions, including dizziness, memory loss, and lack of concentration. Former world chess champion Anatoly Karpov used Professor Buteyko's breathing method to prepare for international chess tournaments. It worked for him by enhancing his concentration.

Panic attacks (see pages 122–125) are severely aggravated by hyperventilation. Reactions can be triggered by activities that sufferers would normally take in their strides, such as crowds, heavy traffic, a congested elevator, or even normal human contact. When you start to panic, you overbreathe even more. This further reduces the oxygen supply to the brain, which in turn increases the panic. Another vicious cycle sets in.

Anxiety, anger, stress, depression, and even agoraphobia (fear of open spaces) are all manifestations of hyperventilation. There may be other, psychological causes behind these states, but overbreathing is an important factor in their severity and recurrence. In many, many cases, physical illnesses disappear when the patient's breathing is rebalanced, and emotional conditions are also righted.

It is important to note that during the Breath Connection program, a few people experience dysfunctional mental states, including anger, irritability, and depression for a short period. This occurs because the body is working hard to rebalance itself. Many therapists would consider this a good sign—in that suppressed emotions are coming out, leaving a clean slate behind. If you feel uncomfortable, or if it becomes a problem, stop the exercises for a few days and start again.

Key Points

- We have learned in this chapter that breathing is not something that only affects our respiratory system, but has an impact on the workings of the entire body.
- Whether or not you suffer from any of the illnesses that can be successfully and directly treated by the Breath Connection program, you can benefit from reconditioned breathing.

Now we are ready to look at how the Breath Connection program can be integrated into every aspect of your daily life.

12

Feeding Your Health

Of all the controversial, almost revolutionary, principles embraced by Breath Connection, those concerning food and diet initiate the most surprise. What we advocate overturns many of the beliefs central to the philosophies of most traditional dieticians and nutritionists, although it is in line with some practices in complementary medicine.

At Breath Connection, we don't even discuss diet with our patients until the second or third day of the program, by which time they will have learned a great deal about how to control their hyperventilation. You can, however, start observing our dietary guidelines from day one.

The system we advise almost always results in a steady balancing of your weight, until your optimum or ideal weight is achieved. That's a happy bonus, as we do not set out to help people slim down or put on much-needed weight. Overweight people invariably lose pounds while following the Breath Connection program. Equally, anorexics and even the slightly underweight find that by following the Breath Connection dietary guidelines as well as the breathing exercises, a correct level of appetite is restored. Some anorexics find that they want to eat small amounts as often as six times a day! By obeying the reeducated calls of a faster metabolism, the body digests food more quickly and more efficiently.

Don't worry about references to timing, such as undertaking exercises before breakfast. If breakfast for you is a cup of herbal tea, that's fine. And don't panic if you have to eat out in a restaurant. Read on to see the wide range of foods you can choose from the menu. Italian, Middle-Eastern, and Indian restaurants may offer the most enticing choices, and they are all within the limits of your program.

It is normally best to stick to vegetarian options in the evening, having your protein meal earlier in the day (see page 191). Be very careful about dairy ingredients that might be included in sauces. Above all, don't feel forced to eat more than you really want, or to try a little taste. For some people, it might be best to avoid eating out during the first few days of the program. This gives the body a chance to adjust to some new habits and nutritional changes.

If the idea of making a dietary change daunts you, have a nice little daydream about something to which you'll treat yourself when the program is complete. Maybe a new piece of clothing in a smaller size? This time next week you can buy it and wear it.

We realize that some individuals may require a customized diet plan and may need to supplement their diets with certain vitamins and minerals. Your Breath Connection practitioner can provide you with a program that will suit your individual needs. The guidelines presented in this section are general ones; if you feel you must adapt them to make it work for you, we suggest you come along to see one of our practitioners, who can give you some good advice.

Mealtimes

Our most important rule is that you should eat only when and if you are hungry. Never eat because it is a certain time of the day; because the people you are with are eating; or because your mother, partner, diet book, or doctor says you should eat. Eat because, and only because, your body tells you it wants food.

Despite its perfect logic, this may not be easy to accept. Most of us were brought up to believe that regular mealtimes were an essential part of good health. We were taught that breakfast is the most important meal of the day, and that skipping it would damage our mental and physical energy. In the first instance, our mothers, shortly followed by endless books and articles on nutrition, stressed that regular fuel was necessary for our bodies to function—particularly while we are young and growing. Apart from anything else, the idea of sitting down with friends and family, and merely sipping water or a fruit drink while they are enjoying a full meal, may not be appealing. It is, however, an essential habit to learn.

Fixed mealtimes have become fixtures, and they were not always devised for our convenience, as anyone who has been roused at 6 A.M. for a hospital breakfast or served an airline lunch at 11 will testify. Don't let other people's schedules dictate yours. Don't eat to please your mother, hostess, or spouse. Listen to your body, and feed it when it tells you that it needs food. If your appetite is fierce at four o'clock in the afternoon, have a proper meal, not just a snack. Arrange things so that you are near a source of good, nutritious food if you are away from home, or pack a suitable picnic in anticipation. Don't feel you need to build yourself up if you are unwell. At such times, your body needs its energy to aid your recovery, not to digest food, particularly if it is the wrong kind of food.

Central to all of this is the fact that eating without hunger makes you hyperventilate and the symptoms of respiratory illness will be aggravated. The very fact that you are opening your mouth and taking in air that way is, of course, a contributing factor.

Good and Bad Foods

We have all been indoctrinated to the fact that we should not eat junk food. It is low in nutrients and normally contains additives, preservatives, sugar, and other chemicals that are all detrimental to good health. These chemicals are toxic and can cause your body to hyperventilate in order to get rid of them. Of course, many natural foods contain toxic substances, but they are in much smaller amounts. Junk food is not to be confused with fast food. You can make delicious and nutritious snacks and meals as quickly as waiting for a pizza delivery to arrive, and you might even save some money. Vegetables, grains, and cereals are inexpensive compared to ready-made foods.

Overeating many foods, such as animal proteins (which include meat, fish, eggs, and milk), increases our intake of breath per minute. Our bodies cannot utilize proteins without first breaking them down into their constituent amino acids. The extra energy required to perform this task—in the form of oxygen—is similar to that needed for a brisk walk of some duration. That's why, after eating a high-protein meal, your breathing becomes labored as your body struggles to digest it. It's also the reason why so many people are sapped of energy after a heavy meal.

As the day progresses, include less and less protein in your diet. It's not a new theory that heavy meals should be avoided late in the evening, but we go a step further. We suggest that not only should you avoid late-night eating, but you should cut down or cut out protein completely in your last meal of the day. A near-certain way to a poor night's sleep—and, of course, hyperventilation—is to eat heavily and unwisely before going to bed. A late protein meal is not only hard on your stomach, which has to work overtime to digest it while you and your body's other systems are trying to rest, but it encourages deep breathing, the very thing we are trying to prevent.

Another received wisdom is that it is good for you to drink as many as eight glasses of water a day. According to Professor Buteyko, you should drink as much water as it takes to quench your thirst. The amounts will vary from person to person.

We do, of course, have a blacklist of forbidden foods. These include such high-protein foods as cheese and other dairy foods, especially milk, yogurt, crème fraîche, goat's cheese, and goat's milk. Apart from being high in protein, dairy foods encourage mucus production, which can be dangerous for an asthmatic. Soy-based foods, chicken, red meat, and fish should also be limited. You (and your child) can obtain calcium from many food sources other than the familiar dairy ones (see page 192). We also advise strongly against the use of table salt, although natural sea salt crystals are fine for seasoning. Steer clear of foods that contain caffeine—and that includes tea, cola drinks, chocolate and cocoa, as well as coffee.

Professor Buteyko found that the foods that contribute to the elimination of asthma and other respiratory illnesses are vegetables—especially green vegetables—and whole grains, such as brown rice. If you are desperate for something milky, try rice milk. Potatoes are also OK in moderation.

If this sounds dreary, you will be heartened to know that Professor Buteyko advocates the use of seasonings such as black pepper, mustard, herbs, onions, and garlic. Use olive oil in cooking, rather than butter, and choose whole-grain bread over processed white or brown. Eat plenty of fresh fruit.

You can eat lamb, chicken, pulses, and fish in moderation, but learn to ditch the notion that a meal isn't proper if it doesn't include protein. Nutritionists agree that an adult should consume an average 20 grams of protein a day, with children and athletes requiring a larger quantity. Those with certain medical conditions may also require a higher amount of protein.

Foods that are high in calcium can also aid sleep and stave off conditions such as osteoporosis. Natural sources include kelp, turnip greens, rhubarb, broccoli, lamb's kidneys, tofu, tinned salmon with bones, baked beans, halibut, fortified oatmeal and other cereals, molasses, all leafy green vegetables, and kale. Don't be fooled into thinking that a glass of milk at mealtimes is necessary; you can get more calcium from other sources than you can from any dairy product.

Mealtime Guidelines

- Try to plan breakfasts consisting of fresh fruit or juices; porridge made with water and served with running honey or pure maple syrup; cereals with rice milk; toast with an olive oil spread; a bowl of mixed seeds, nuts, and dried fruit; or a cereal bar.
- Lunch could consist of a small amount of lamb, chicken, or fish, with a salad and some lightly cooked veg-

etables. You could choose a baked potato or rice with vegetables very sparingly drizzled with virgin olive oil. For dessert, try a fresh fruit sorbet or some nondairy cake. Fruit salad (without cream, of course!) is ideal.

• At dinnertime (or, indeed, earlier in the day), you could have some pasta or noodles with a tomato or pesto sauce, or any of the nonprotein options that were offered for your previous meal. Roast or steamed Mediterranean vegetables can be delicious, and they are extremely healthy.

• Follow the rules of any responsible diet and cut out processed foods. Alcohol is also a toxin, and should, if possible, be avoided in the early stages of the program.

• Try to eat slowly, chewing properly, with your mouth closed.

• Leave food on the side of your plate when you have had enough.

• Shop thoughtfully and study labels for additives and hidden sugars.

• Eat organic, which is much healthier—and tastier!

• If you can, buy as much as possible from health and whole-food shops. It may prove to be a little more expensive, but you can eat and enjoy your meal with confidence.

• It is also better to shop ahead, so you won't be tempted to grab something unsuitable from the nearest outlet when hunger strikes. It's a good idea to have some healthy cereal snacks on hand at all times.

Diet Checklist

• Eat only when you are hungry.
• Do not overeat.
• Try to avoid high-protein foods.
• Avoid caffeine.

- Reduce your sugar intake.
- Avoid milk in any form, except rice milk.
- Avoid cheese, yogurt, and other dairy products.
- Eat plenty of whole grains and fresh green vegetables.
- Use natural sea salt, not table salt.
- Drink water when you are thirsty, but not unless you are.
- Listen to your body's demands and don't be bullied into eating by other people.

No significant dietary change is easy. It may be even harder to change a child's eating habits. Be positive, and tell your child that it won't be long before he or she experiences the benefits of an altered diet. Children adapt easily, and they soon forget old routines. Before long, the new program will be the norm, and your child may well prefer it to the old one. Tears at mealtimes are easier to cope with than asthma attacks in the night, so bear that in mind when your child objects to the fact that creamy chocolate sponge cake is no longer on the menu.

Your own progress and that of your children will advance almost exponentially if you all follow the dietary guidelines we have outlined here.

13

Planning and Preparation

Any major life change has the potential to be energizing and exciting. It makes sense, however, to anticipate the doubts, worries, and even fears that naturally accompany any break from the familiar. It often takes a great leap of faith, and considerable confidence, to make permanent changes in our lives, whether those changes affect our relationships, our work, or our home life. Changes to our health can be positive, but it is not unusual for people to feel hesitant about committing to a new lifestyle, particularly if they felt confident and secure in the old one.

In this chapter, we show you how choosing to adopt the Breath Connection way of life is easy. With a little thought and planning, it can be so enjoyable, you may wonder why you ever delayed.

At times, all of us cling to the security blanket of our bad habits, or even illnesses. Habits and states of mind and health supply us with part of our identity. It is an interesting phenomenon that human beings tend to set themselves up for failure, no matter how much the results are coveted. Although we may realize, intellectually, that a change is for the best—whether it involves changing the way we look, how much we weigh, our overall health, or all three—it is often difficult to put that longing for change into action. You know the feeling: Perhaps you have tried lots of self-improvement courses or treatments, such as diets, skincare regimes, exercise routines, only to have failed to commit to or fulfill your ambitions. Perhaps you dread the challenge of new opportunities that a new and improved self might have to face.

It's important to remind yourself—and do so constantly—that there is never really any new self. That healthier and more confident person is still you, and you are someone who can now familiarize yourself with your new potential.

There are a few logical preliminaries to consider before embarking on the Breath Connection program. Being realistic and honest with yourself will help to make the program work for you—and with you. Here is some practical advice:

• Make practical preparations. Arrange a conducive environment for your exercises. If you can't designate a separate room where you can be alone for short periods throughout the day, screen off a corner of the bedroom or a seldom-used room such as a dining room, if you have one.

• Elicit outside support. Tell everyone who interacts with you on a daily basis what you are doing and why. Anyone who cares about you is bound to be encouraging. Moreover, it is undoubtedly more difficult to lapse, let alone fail, if you have stated your aims. A sense of pride, or the feeling that you are letting others down, can help to keep you motivated.

• Develop a positive mental attitude. You can motivate yourself by the promise of a treat or a night out with friends, if you keep to the program for a week. Promise another, special, reward for when you reach your goal.

- Anticipate obstacles in advance, and plan for them. Have a contingency plan for days when you can't seem to find time to be alone, or you just couldn't exercise as you'd planned. This isn't being negative, just pragmatic.

- Be realistic and recognize that it is human nature to procrastinate. This doesn't give you carte blanche to do so, but you won't feel so discouraged when the temptation to put things off is at its most appealing.

- It is also human nature to want results without having to work for them. Don't castigate yourself for giving in to such thoughts. Not *very* deep down you know that little is achieved in any field without some effort and discipline. Just remind yourself that any major change involves time, energy, and a little bit of enthusiasm. In your case, it may also involve the sacrifice of some favorite foods or giving up the habit of eating a late dinner. Remind yourself that these small losses will soon be dismissed as you learn new and better habits. Visualize the healthy, freer life you will have when you complete the course. If that visualization includes an improved appearance, so much the better. Visualize yourself having the energy to participate in games with your children, to play a sport, or to dance with your friends in a way that has been restricted until now. Visualize yourself free from artificial drugs, allowing your body to heal itself with its own natural resources. All of these images should not only be very motivating, but, in their way, self-perpetuating. There is no doubt that people with a positive outlook attract positive energies in life, and the reverse is also true. You can make it happen. These positive affirmations and mental rehearsals can strengthen your resolve. The Breath Connection exercises are not so lengthy or strenuous that much steely resolve should be necessary. Results are quick and effective, and you will, in turn, be motivated by the speed at which you see change.

• Don't be ill any longer than you have to be. You should be aware that you will receive the care, attention, and sympathy of your loved ones whether you are healthy or not. Friends and family will be so delighted by your recovery that you will receive just as much attention. Their attention may be a little less deferential and solicitous, but it will be based on an equal footing, rather than a carer-to-invalid relationship. Isn't that preferable?

Deciding that you want to change your health, your habits, and, through that, your life, is the first vital leg of the Breath Connection voyage. It does, however, need to be supported by a practical strategy, something that has been designed to work for you and your individual circumstances. This is partly why we keep stressing that although we believe that all readers can gain and learn from our book, sometimes the special attention of a qualified practitioner can make the little bit of difference that can push you that extra half mile.

The following practical preparations are for the average reader and should work in the majority of cases. Take care to read and work through them all. They are likely to meet all of your particular needs, especially if you tweak things a little here and there to allow them to fit your lifestyle.

If you can, check your schedule before embarking on the course and try to block off short times of the day or evening, two, three, or four times a day. Many people respond well to the discipline of fulfilling commitments that have been arranged. Make a date with yourself to practice Breath Connection, and reserve that time as yours. Give this date the same priority that you would any engagement, and don't break it unless you have to.

Practical Preparation

The Breath Connection program should initially be followed two to four times a day for a minimum of five days. Different sections of this book address the treatment of various ailments, and offer specific advice on how often, and for how long, you can expect to exercise. Do bear in mind that regularity and consistency are important when following the program, and if you earmark special times of the day for your exercises, it will make a substantial difference. This means advance planning. Where are you going to exercise? At home, in the office, in the gym? Think about the week you have selected to start the Breath Connection program and plan accordingly, postponing nonessential dates if necessary. Remember that you will only need a few minutes for each session, which should, ideally, take place first thing in the morning, just before lunch, before your evening meal, and just before bed. If you find it difficult to fit it all in, start your program in a quieter, less socially demanding week in the near future. Once you have your program in place, you'll find it easier to find time to fit it in—particularly since you will have seen the results and feel more motivated.

If you need to make new arrangements, always fit them in around your Breath Connection commitments. Remember that you have made an appointment with yourself and it is your priority. We are aware that people with demanding jobs, in the office or in a household with children, for example, may find it difficult to make and keep to commitments. Many of us are used to putting ourselves second, or even third, while we cope with busy jobs or family life. In order for you to experience good health, you need to take care of yourself. That means learning to put yourself first and ensuring that your priorities are right. You always have time for the things you put first.

It's equally important that people with less demanding lifestyles make a date and stick to it. If you have a long, empty day stretching ahead of you, it's easy to rationalize that you have all the time in the world, and that you will fit in your exercises at some point. Chances are, however, that the day will slip by and you won't ever get to them. Make an appointment with yourself and treat it as a priority.

Environment

The place where you practice your Breath Connection exercise should, ideally, be quiet, private, comfortable, and warm. If there is a telephone nearby, disconnect it for those few minutes and enjoy the added luxury of silence. If your household is a bustling one, you might like to hang a "do not disturb" sign on the door of your chosen place, for the short duration of the exercises. Explain to your family what you are doing, and request a few moments' peace.

We know that some people have become so captivated by the Breath Connection process that they have redecorated the rooms in which they practice in tranquil colors to suit the mood. Excellent! Of course, we realize that this is not practical for everyone, but it does help to practice in an inspiring environment. Some people have created an environment in which they will work best by surrounding themselves with a few favorite objects or pictures. Make your space as positive and inspiring as you possibly can. You should never feel that you are shoved into a corner. This is your time, and your space. You want to feel comfortable and relaxed. This is quality time, aimed at improving your health on every level. Make sure you create an atmosphere that is conducive to that.

Time-Keeping

You will need an accurate clock, with a second hand. Better still, invest in a stopwatch to count your Control Pause with accuracy. Purchase some micropore tape (see page 51), and keep it on hand for use when you are alone in the house.

Diet

Plan your meals for the week and shop in advance, ensuring that there are no forbidden foods in the refrigerator to tempt you during moments of weakness. We talk more about diet in Chapter 12 (see pages 190–194). Buy a few healthy but delicious snacks from health food shops if you fear the odd emergency. Inform your family or partner of your new routine, and ask him or her for support. The main idea is to eat only when you are hungry. Others may have to get used to you being at the table without eating.

Try to avoid a high-protein meal in the evening (see page 191), and avoid foods with additives, or anything that has been processed. Dairy foods are also not recommended, so you will need to create delicious and nutritious meals based on fruits, vegetables, and a wonderful range of carbohydrates. Eat fish, meat, and pulses only in moderation.

If you must travel for business or pleasure while you are following the Breath Connection program, phone the airline and order a vegetarian or vegan meal. This is particularly important for diagnosed asthmatics or emphysemics, as a heavy protein meal in cabin conditions will aggravate breathing difficulties.

If you forget to book a meal in advance, pack your own snack or drink water on the journey and save your appetite for your arrival at your destination. It can be difficult to avoid, particularly if you are traveling on business, or even pleasure, but try not to eat out during the first few days of your course. If it is unavoidable, tell friends that you are on a restricted diet and explain why you are doing so. Most restaurants have fresh salads and delicious vegetarian options. Stick with these while you are eating out. Try to remember Professor Buteyko's advice about eating only when you are hungry and not because it is mealtime. You can socialize perfectly well at a dinner as you pick at a suitable salad.

The best thing you can eat late at night is a plate of vegetables, and some complex carbohydrates, such as a whole grain or brown rice or potatoes. It can be difficult to watch friends or family digging into steaming and fragrant heaps of your favorite foods, but try to remember that this regime will not continue indefinitely. Perhaps you can persuade some like-minded friends to join you in your special diet.

Replace ordinary salt with crunchier mineral salt. Tea and coffee are not villains, but try to drink them as infrequently as possible, and without milk or cream. Herbal teas are particularly refreshing, or try something such as roasted dandelion root coffee, which is naturally creamy and much healthier. If you feel frustrated, inspire yourself with the promise of a special treat—such as an evening out, or a new piece of clothing—at the end of the program. Try to make yourself feel pampered and not deprived. Buy a book that you have been longing for, or invest in a new CD. Surround yourself with special treats and you won't feel the bite of change.

It is also important to cut down on alcohol during the Breath Connection program. Although it will, at first, help you shallow breathe, it eventually leads to overbreathing. You might be interested to know that this is one of the main causes of hangovers. It can be difficult to resist alcohol when you are socializing, which is why it is important to begin the program during a quiet week. Some people enjoy a drink at the end of the day, to help them to relax or sleep. If you fall into this category, try to keep yourself busy so that you are tired enough to want to turn in and sleep when you get home.

Your body will adapt to the revised eating plan very quickly, and, in a short time, will not expect to be fueled at the old, regular times.

Exercise

For those of you who have exercise or other sports commitments, it may be unnecessary to make some changes to your regular routine while on the Breath Connection program. Just remember to keep your mouth closed, and be aware of the way you breathe as you exercise. This is particularly important for swimmers. Remember not to open your mouth to take in air when you reach the surface. Breathe through your nose at all times. Do a Control Pause before and after exercise, and if your score is less than 20 seconds, give yourself a break from that particular sport until your breath is regulated.

Never deep breathe after any type of exercise. This may seem like an impossibility now, but once you have started the Breath Connection program, you will find it easier and easier to achieve. Once you have taught yourself to breathe shallowly as an automatic response, you will not find it hard to continue breathing in this way, even after strenuous activity.

Asthmatics should be careful to avoid any activity for which they currently use a bronchodilator. This indicates that there is body resistance to the exercise, and you should listen to the message that your body is giving you. Remember that you are in brief and life-changing training for a short period of time, and you should do your best to be in prime condition before beginning the Breath Connection program.

Eliciting Outside Support

The power and support of friends, family, and organized groups cannot be overstated. Gamblers and Alcoholics Anonymous and Weight Watchers, among others, all testify to the role that caring people can play in helping someone break a bad habit or addiction. The first step is often the most difficult one—that of telling people that you have a problem and would like their encouragement as you set about solving it. Women are, in general, more likely to enlist outside support than men, but everyone on the Breath Connection program should have someone with whom they can talk things through. Don't be afraid to ask for help.

Cancer patients have had their life expectancies doubled when they have support groups to lean on, or even one special person to help share the strain. Heart bypass patients have also been shown to benefit from talking things through with groups of fellow sufferers, particularly if there is a measure of good humor involved.

Fortunately, with Breath Connection there is no stigma to overcome. People are not, in general, judgmental, and you will find that your determination to make changes will inspire encouragement. If necessary, ask your employer to be understanding and to tolerate occasional late arrivals in the morning, and short periods of the day when you will need to concentrate on your exercises. By overcoming any respiratory illness, and encouraging your body to work at peak level, your professional performance will be enhanced—a fact that can't hesitate to win over even the most skeptical boss.

Show this book to friends and colleagues, and explain what you want to achieve. Tell them that you are going to follow the Breath Connection program and ask for their encouragement. Don't be daunted if a few people are negative or even amused. We are used to cynicism here, and there will always be people who scoff at the idea that it is possible to make broad-scale health changes by altering the way you breathe. You may even find people who provide you with tales of the importance of deep breathing. Turn away from these doubters and be strong in your conviction. Follow the good instincts that led you to Breath Connection in the first place.

In the first week, try to avoid all who have been negative or unsupportive. If this isn't possible, ask them to respect what you are trying to do, just as you can respect their differing views. You need to be able to focus your energy on the program and should avoid anyone or any situation that threatens your wholehearted commitment.

Most important, remember that in five days your results will speak for themselves. If you do have any lingering doubts about embarking on the program, be positive with yourself and play up the potential gains more than the challenges. After all, what have you got to lose? By investing only five days to begin with, you will experience changes that can transform the way you think and feel.

It is particularly helpful to begin the program with someone else. Naturally, your partner or friend is unlikely to have exactly the same health conditions that you do, but your partner is bound to benefit from the program even if he or she feels completely well. It is more fun to have a friend to compare notes with, and it's important that there is someone to offer strong support if you feel like giving up.

Positive Mental Attitude

Are you someone who sees a glass as being half full or half empty? Are you a pessimist or an optimist? We encourage optimism and believe that concentrating on the potential gains of following the program rather than the negative aspects—giving up a favorite food, for example—will make a huge difference to your overall success. Dietary changes are a drawback for a number of people who begin the program, but we can assure you that the changes you need to make are minor. You will be eating well, and as much as you want to. You won't be sacrificing much at all. Be positive about your commitment and you will reap the rewards.

The decision you made to commit to the Breath Connection program was an enormous stride in the right direction. Some people find it helpful to see visual reminders of the healthy outcome of their course—pictures of people enjoying the pleasures of life, such as taking a long walk in the country, or playing an active sport with friends. Try to choose a picture of an activity in which you see yourself participating when the program is complete. If you are hoping to lose some weight, pin up a picture of an article of clothing that you want to fit into when your weight is regulated. If you suffer from disturbed sleep, find a photograph of someone enjoying a deep and peaceful sleep. Your motivation will be unique to you, and you will need to decide what will work best.

Some people respond to spoken motivation. Tapes offering calm, steady encouragement are available for you to listen to in the comfort of your home. We don't recommend that you play them while driving, as you need to remain alert while you are behind the wheel.

We know that the mind has a very powerful role to play in all self-healing situations. The mind-body relationship is a strong one, and literally hundreds of studies have proven that fact. When you feel good emotionally, you are more likely to feel well physically. Sports professionals psyche themselves up before major competitions, and allow their positive attitude to improve their performance. You can aid your own success by telling yourself, or showing yourself, how much better things will be when you complete the course. Our minds do not differentiate between an activity that is actually taking place and one that is simply and realistically imagined. Take advantage of the powers of mental rehearsal by visualizing your body as strong, healthy, and less drug-dependent.

Make a list of all the positive results you expect to achieve by the end of the five-day course. Make a collage with pictures and words cut from magazines, if they make a contribution to the picture you have of yourself when you are at your best. Perhaps you still have a photograph of yourself, taken when you were in peak health, to remind you. Indulge in a little fantasy of a dream holiday. Go on imaginary shopping sprees. Remind yourself that you might just be a little closer to your wish list if you persevere with the Breath Connection course.

Working Out Obstacles

One of the best ways to overcome obstacles is to anticipate them, and to plan how they will be confronted or circumvented. However carefully you have prepared for the course, and however firm your intentions are, you will undoubtedly face a setback at some stage. The important thing is not to be discouraged. Don't imagine that you are the first or only person to experience a glitch in your program. So you didn't meet your Control Pause target one day? It's not a tragedy, and you shouldn't even consider giving up.

Note down things that might go wrong. Maybe one day you will be interrupted in midexercise and will not have the time to start again. How will you deal with that? Perhaps you gave in to sleeping on your right side because you have always found that position more natural and more comfortable. Maybe you couldn't resist a big, frothy cappuccino. Think back to situations when you have broken your resolve in the past—early in the New Year, for example. Try to remember why you lapsed. Chances are that you weren't ready to change your bad habit. Now you are. You have committed to the Breath Connection course, and the very fact that you mind so much about a small setback proves that you are still committed to it.

If you fall off the horse, climb back on. Don't chastise yourself for slips. Accept that it is human nature to give in every now and then, and congratulate yourself for starting again, with a renewed effort.

Above all, be fair to yourself. Remember that you have embarked on a program of huge change. To reduce your drug intake in only five days is an enormous achievement, especially if you are a severe asthmatic. Congratulate yourself for the progress you have made, and avoid tormenting yourself for any imperfections. Years of being instructed to breathe deeply mean that some people may take longer than five days to achieve the target. That doesn't mean you have failed.

Take your time, think of something inspirational, and get back to work.

Sometimes we call inspiration a compelling outcome, and there can be any number of these, such as better digestion, improved sleep, freedom from drugs, social confidence, ideal weight, freedom from the fear of an attack, or even just an enhanced sense of well-being. Just thinking about any one of these goals should help to get you back on track. It is admirable to have high standards, but setting your sights too high means that you have further to fall when things do not go according to plan. Be realistic, and don't let your disappointment lead to dejection. Remember that you are doing amazingly well, considering what you have had to overcome.

The Appeal of Procrastination

Most people who habitually procrastinate abominate this tendency in themselves. A lucky few genuinely embrace the *mañana* philosophy of life, and actually believe that troubles will disappear if you ignore them for long enough. But the majority of procrastinators are guilt-ridden perfectionists who know perfectly well that tiresome tasks are best faced sooner rather than later, but who delay for a variety of reasons. One common reason for procrastination is the fear of success. Many people fear that they will not accomplish a task as well as their standards demand, and rather than suffer the indignity or disappointment of failure, they do not even begin.

If you have been thinking about the Breath Connection program but continue to put it off, just remember how empowering, how triumphant it feels to address a project over which you have been dithering. Tell other people what you plan. You are more likely to stick with something that you have made grand pronouncements about. Not many of us will suffer the loss of face involved in publicly giving up. The more people you tell, the harder it will be to quit. But be realistic, and don't book yourself onto a course that you will find difficult to complete. If you are changing jobs, having a baby, getting married, or moving to another house, you might want to delay things until your life is a little more settled.

If you continue to put off the Breath Connection program, even though intellectually and in every other way you know it makes sense, perhaps you should consider whether you are clinging to your illness, or present state of being, because its familiarity makes you feel secure. Your physical and emotional conditions are part of your identity, and it isn't always easy to change something so fundamental. Look hard at yourself. If you think the reasons for your failure to begin are linked with this type of attitude, accept them and use that self-knowledge to spur you on. If you are worried about the new challenges that life will impose on you when you are strong and healthy again, think positively. This is going to be the start of a fantastic adventure, something that will soon seem much more appealing than the comfortable cocoon of fearful habit. Acknowledging your fear is the first step to overcoming it, and we can help you do that.

Wanting Results Without Work

Another common human trait is our tendency to want something for nothing. We want results without effort. In our daydreams, we may have perfect looks, perfect health, perfect homes, jobs, and lives. . . . These are healthy inspirational images, and you should hang on to them when you start the Breath Connection program. Just bear in mind that only so much is realistic. We are sure you know very few people who have all of the preceding, and if they do, it is likely that they have worked very hard to achieve that status. Don't expect to gain anything without giving it some effort. Commit yourself to the program, and welcome the change it brings. The certainty is that you will be nearer to achieving what you want when your breathing has been reconditioned.

This is the reality: It is going to take some effort. Stay where you are, with your daydreams and your deteriorating health, or take control and make some effort to effect permanent change. Athletes who want to break records need dedication. So do students who want to achieve the highest honors. If you truly want to experience the benefits of balanced breathing, and the changes that this will bring, you have to work at it. We promise that the effort will soon become second nature and, as such, effortless.

Never say that you don't have time. All of us can make time for the things that matter, and as we said earlier, we always have time for the things we put first. Breath Connection involves committing to just a few minutes, three or four times a day. Your renewed zest for life will allow you to do things more quickly and efficiently, and you will sleep better, and for shorter periods, as a result. Spending a little time now will actually buy you some time later. And time wasted in doctors' or hospital waiting rooms will be a thing of the past. The Breath Connection program will be giving you more time—years and years of it.

Remember the old adage: You need to speculate to accumulate. By investing time today in the Breath Connection program, you will have achieved more than you could ever have imagined. That means a longer, healthier, freer life. Isn't it worth it?

14

The Maintenance Plan

Our plan begins with five days of your time. Not every hour of five days, but a few minutes, every so often. In this extraordinarily short space of time, an entire lifetime of harmful breathing can be adjusted and reconditioned. The path toward health and well-being can be paved.

You have already invested your time and effort, and even if you were to stop right now, your enterprise would have been well worthwhile. The changes that you will have already observed in your breathing, sleeping, susceptibility to asthma, and other attacks are remarkable. But now that your engine has been so thoroughly overhauled, and its performance is so dramatically better, don't you want to keep up the momentum and continue to improve? Aren't you keen to build on your achievement? At the very least, it makes sense to embark on a maintenance plan that will ensure your new energy is sustained.

Some Breath Connection patients are confident enough to enter the next phases of their lives without fear of relapse. Others continue to follow the self-care program we supply. Still others, those with more severe conditions, benefit from the continued supervision of a Breath Connection practitioner. It would be tragic if any of the good work achieved during those first, crucial five days were wasted, so we continue to offer encouragement when it is needed.

If you are concerned that you might not be disciplined enough to keep up the good work, you might need to continue to monitor your breathing habits after the five-day course. For all Breath Connection practitioners, retrained shallow breathing is second nature, so they do not need to set aside time for Control Pauses and pulse readings, unless they happen to be feeling unwell. For you to reach this level of confidence, you should continue with the exercises for a little while after the course. Eventually, shallow, retrained breathing will become completely automatic. If a stressful period comes along, and you think you may lapse into hyperventilating, it is reassuring to know that you can deal with it by reverting to the regular and, by now, familiar exercises. Emphysemic, bronchial, or asthmatic attacks can be a thing of the past.

The fast and dramatic improvements that all patients experience over the five-day course are, of course, a great incentive to keep going. For people with severe respiratory or other health problems, the success achieved in those first days will be all the motivation they need to continue. Expert help at the outset will always be useful for more seriously ill patients to look after themselves in the future.

Our maintenance program has been designed to fit into most people's modern lifestyles. It is also based on a sort of bond of trust. We assume that patients are not going to slip immediately back into the bad habits that lead them to us in the first place. Equally, we know that you do not expect us to make you instantly well after a lapse, a stressful period, or an illness, and you are aware that Breath Connection is not a miracle pill or a wonder drug. What we can do is improve your overall health to such a degree that illness is quickly and efficiently dealt with.

It's important to remember that you should never push yourself beyond comfortable limits. This program isn't about competition, even with yourself. However delighted you may be to see your Control Pause reach 60, and however much you may be feeling the benefits of correct breathing, you do not need to continue to push beyond that point. You have achieved a personal best! If you wish to develop your Control Pause above 60, this must be done under the supervision of a Breath Connection practitioner. This method is very powerful and you will need expert guidance if you wish to improve your breathing performance further.

Take stock after completing your five-day course and do the following:

- Recognize how much more healthy you feel.
- Continue to eliminate some of the physical threats in your life by maintaining your retrained breathing, sleeping, and eating patterns.
- Do all you can to prevent or remove triggers that may cause future illness.
- Build on what you have already achieved to expand your potential for good health.

Practical Advice

The most essential thing is to keep up your shallow breathing. If you need to be reminded, put notes around your home or office. It should, however, be more natural by now, and you should still continue to be aware of your breathing patterns throughout the day. If you start breathing deeply again, immediately change to shallow breathing.

Keep your mouth shut unless you are talking, eating, or drinking—wherever you are. Keep up the habit of placing tape on your mouth before you go to sleep at night. This practice can be discontinued if you are absolutely certain that you are no longer breathing through your mouth while asleep, but until that time, the tape is a good safeguard. Be especially watchful if you find you are snoring again, or if your mouth is dry in the morning.

Continue to sleep on your left side propped up by pillows, to ensure that you do not lose too much carbon dioxide. It's impossible to offer a reason why this works, but years of empirical research by Professor Buteyko have confirmed that sleeping upright, propped up against pillows on your left-hand side, can help to ensure the proper balance of carbon dioxide and oxygen in your body.

Stick to the diet recommended in Chapter 12. Above all, don't eat a heavy protein meal at night (see page 191). Keep dairy foods and sugars to a minimum, and continue to avoid processed and junk foods as much as possible. By now you may have lost your craving for them. Many people will have found that they want to eat much less at mealtimes. Keep up the good work!

Exercise as much as is practical and sensible, and remember to keep your mouth closed when doing so. Remember that the mechanism for your breathing is located in your brain, and the more you practice shallow breathing, the more automatic it will become. Any new behavior or action needs to be practiced consciously before it becomes an unconscious act, and it is particularly vital that you practice until it does become instinctive. You will prevent a lifetime of suffering and disease and feel better than you would ever have believed possible as a result.

Check your pulse and Control Pause every single day, in order to monitor your breathing progress as well as your overall health. If you can, try to see a Breath Connection practitioner from time to time in order to get expert advice if your health has changed in any way. Never try to push your Control Pause when you are on your own. This is a powerful treatment, and it must not be done for too long. Just as you would take no more than a couple of pain relievers when you have a headache, you must treat the Control Pause with respect.

Now that you are working on your own, try not to become overconfident or reckless with your exercises. On the other hand, don't feel that you have failed in any way if you need to see a practitioner for guidance.

Maintenance Suggestions for Mild Asthma

Carry on with the self-care program (see page 79) until you are able to manage without bronchodilators. Maintain your Control Pause at the level it was when you stopped using these drugs. Never, ever push it beyond comfortable limits in the interest of getting a result. This is both counterproductive and dangerous. Your reduced steroid intake should be supervised by your doctor in conjunction with a Breath Connection expert. Don't stop taking your steroids altogether, or you risk a relapse. If you are eventually able to cut them out entirely, it will only be after a slow and steady withdrawal.

Maintenance Suggestions for Severe Asthma

Follow the self-care program on page 93 on a daily basis, but adapt it when your severe asthma becomes mild. Then follow the guidelines recommended for steroid intake (see pages 67–72).

Maintenance Guidelines for Emphysema and Bronchitis
Emphysemics should continue with the program indefinitely. Those with bronchitis should follow it until the bronchitis disappears. If you still feel there is cause for concern, don't hesitate to see your Breath Connection counselor again. Then, continue with self-care.

Maintenance Guidelines for Sports Maintenance
Check your Control Pause before and after any sporting activity and keep your mouth closed for its duration. Before exercise, practice a Control Pause followed by five minutes of shallow breathing. After your exercise, do a Control Pause, followed by five minutes of shallow breathing. Repeat.

There are special chapters in this book offering advice for readers who seek more detailed information about maintenance plans for asthmatic children (see page 149), people prone to panic attacks (see page 124), and for overall, holistic good health (see page 134).

Do I Really Want to Feel Well Again?
Of course you do. All of us would like to experience the type of good health that others take for granted. Perhaps, however, something is holding you back from building upon the good work you have achieved over the five-day course. Perhaps you are under stress, and adhering to our guidelines seems like one more pressure. Many people suffering from stress find it difficult to make changes; clinging to what they perceive to be the few rocks of certainty in their lives is one way to feel more secure. In order to get well, however, things have to change. Don't be tempted to stick with a situation that is making you stressed. Think of your situation as a rut out of which you can climb. You need to make changes to

climb out, and you need determination. Just as you need the will to be well.

Lacking Motivation?

When you embarked on the Breath Connection program, you had the determination to make change. You can recover that will, even if a state of helplessness, which certainly requires less energy, has its appeal. Use your considerable will to help you to get back on course, and to climb out of that rut.

Remember how frightening asthma attacks were—that pain in your chest and the struggle for every breath? Either you continue to make changes in your life or you face going back to that. If you are in a stressful situation and find it difficult, think positively. Use friends and family for support and advice. Draw on others for motivation, and use as many positive affirmations as you can to keep things moving.

If you are feeling stressed and finding it difficult to motivate yourself, there are some excellent tapes that you can listen to in a quiet, calm place.

Again, don't castigate yourself for a brief loss of purpose. Visualize your ultimate aim and, if you must, visualize yourself at your most damaged state in the past. These visualizations will inspire you again.

15

Question Time

The fact that we are asked some questions over and over again confirms the fact that certain issues and aspects of the Breath Connection program consistently baffle a range of people. We don't like confusion, and we certainly don't mind addressing your questions as many times as it takes for the program to become clear. Here are the most frequently asked questions and the answers we always give.

How should we breathe—from the top of the lungs, the middle, or the bottom?

The way you breathe is less important than the amount of air you take in, as this is what affects the balance of oxygen and carbon dioxide in the lungs. We recommend shallow breathing from the top of the lungs, as this is the best way to avoid hyperventilation.

How many times should I practice the exercises each day?

We advise three to four times a day: early in the morning before breakfast (perform them even if you don't eat breakfast), before lunch, and again before dinner. Do them again about an hour before bed, if you can manage it. If you have regular colds or flu, you can step that up to five or more times a day. Or, if you have a good Control Pause of 30 seconds or more, once or twice a day will be enough.

Why do some people have a low Control Pause but no asthma?

If you hyperventilate and have a low Control Pause, it may be that your body simply chooses to exhibit another defense mechanism to stop you from exhaling too much carbon dioxide. Some of the common diseases associated with hyperventilation include epilepsy, emphysema, diabetes, heart problems, cancer, and other fatal illnesses. Less seriously, snoring and a chronically blocked nose are common symptoms. The fact that your target area is the respiratory system, resulting in asthma, indicates that things are not as bad as they might be. The strain of hyperventilation will always be expressed in the body's weakest area or system. If you have been genetically bestowed with a strong respiratory system, you will not have asthma even if you overbreathe. But if your digestive system is weak, you will experience digestive complaints. If your immune system is weak, you will be more prone to infection.

Do all asthmatics hyperventilate and have a low Control Pause?

Yes. The more severe your asthma, the lower your Control Pause.

What is Salbutamol?

Salbutamol is the generic name for Ventolin.

Why do yoga teachers recommend deep breathing?

Yoga teaches breath control and some exercises might involve either deep or shallow breathing, or holding the breath for a designated period of time. Therefore, Yogic breathing does not always involve hyperventilation. Some yoga teachers have embraced the Western view that deep breathing is good for you. We do not agree with that. The diagram below compares balanced breathing, with lung ventilation of about five liters a minute, with full Yogic breathing. In this type of breathing, very deep, slow breaths are taken and held before exhalation. The person is not taking in huge quantities of air because the breath is drawn so slowly,

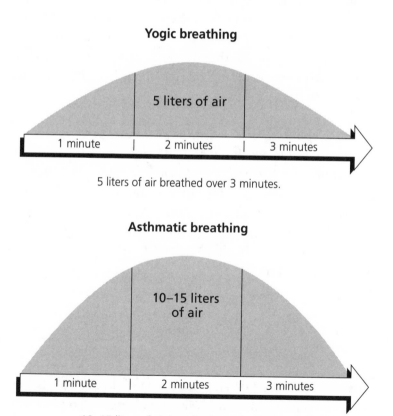

Yogic breathing

5 liters of air

| 1 minute | 2 minutes | 3 minutes |

5 liters of air breathed over 3 minutes.

Asthmatic breathing

10–15 liters of air

| 1 minute | 2 minutes | 3 minutes |

10–15 liters of air breathed over 3 minutes.

with the mouth closed. Yoga has helped some asthmatics, but the results tend to be slow.

I am a yoga teacher and I have mild asthma. What should I do?

Stop deep breathing during yoga exercises and tell your pupils you have done so. Ancient yogis did not have a word for *oxygen* and did recommend breath control, but not as a life pattern, only as an exercise. Deep breathing would not be recommended for asthmatics. In fact, your deep breathing may have caused your asthma. Remember that deep breathing has only ever been a part of a yogic program, not something to practice constantly, any more than you would follow another yogic exercise such as remaining balanced on your head for 24 hours a day.

I am a telephonist/teacher with moderate asthma and I have to talk a lot at work. What should I do?

Follow the Breath Connection program and improve your Control Pause. The lower your Control Pause, the more you will find it difficult to talk and the more you will hyperventilate. Learn to talk from your lips only, not taking deep breaths before you begin. Moderate your breath between pauses. You will probably have to take a little more time to relay your message.

I am an extremely busy businessperson, and I have severe asthma. What steps should I take?

You should try to get away from your professional stresses for a week or two. Work on making your asthma mild. If you can take an even longer break, your asthma will become extremely mild if you follow the Breath Connection program. If neither of these options is realistic—although you should think carefully about the ultimate value of your health, and remember that you will be no good to your company if you become seriously debilitated—discuss things with an enlightened doctor, increase your oral steroids in consultation with your doctor, get better exercise, and practice shallow breathing in the airplane or in the back of your car, and during meetings. Steroids could be increased before difficult meetings, during bad weather, and before travel, but do not forget to normalize the dosage when you feel better. Learn how to control your breath when you give talks and presentations (see above). Sleep less, with your mouth taped, so that you will have more time for the exercises. Cut back on alcohol and eat less at business lunches. Have a light, nonprotein meal for business dinners. If you suddenly feel stressed during the day, do a Control Pause and shallow breathe for about three minutes. Smoke less.

I'm a stay-at-home mom with mild asthma, and I have a family of young children. What can I do?

You probably don't think you have time for the Breath Connection exercises, but you do. Like the preceding businessperson, you can make time. When you are enjoying much more restful sleep, it will become easier and easier to do so. Think of all the other things that you struggle to find the time and energy to complete—shopping, cleaning, cooking, collecting children, school activities. You have to breathe, no matter what, so there is no reason not to do it properly. There must be times when you have a few moments to relax and concentrate on your exercises and Control Pause. At the hairdresser? While your children are watching a video? When you are sitting in the garden? In a traffic jam? In the bath? At the very least, train yourself to be aware of your breathing at all times throughout the day.

When we are measuring the Control Pause, why do we empty the lungs rather than hold the breath after breathing in?

It is very important to hold your breath only after you have breathed out. This is particularly important for people with asthma, emphysema, and bronchitis. After you breathe out, your bronchial tubes expand. After breathing in, they narrow. By holding your breath after breathing in, you could develop emphysema through overstretching your lung tissue, and the condition could become aggravated if you already have it. The Control Pause should only ever be measured after breathing out. Holding your breath after breathing in only focuses on your lung capacity, not your degree of overbreathing—and that is what we are aiming to measure.

Do the health conditions you have outlined for the length of the Control Pause apply to both adults and children?

Yes. Age, height, or body size have no effect on the Control Pause. Lung capacity is not an issue.

Why do we need such large lungs if we are supposed to breathe shallowly?

We have a large stomach capacity, even though it isn't strictly necessary. It helps our digestive system to function well. The stomach does not need to be stuffed for this, and it should not be. The stomach was once a reservoir for food when we were hunters. Evolution has outstripped some of the functions of a large stomach, but it still handles the digestive system pretty well. Perhaps we needed that extra capacity for air in our lungs, long ago when people needed more air for the lives they led. Why do we still have the redundant appendix? In a few million years, this organ will probably disappear. It took a long time for humans, whose ancestors came from the sea, to lose their gills. A very few people still have them!

With the self-care program, what kind of improvement can the average asthmatic hope to achieve?

We estimate that the average improvement is about 60 percent reduction in the need for medication, a significant alleviation of asthma symptoms, and a correspondingly more comfortable and enjoyable life. Remember that this is an average figure. If your original situation was desperate, it may take time to reach that level of improvement. If it was only mild or average, the gain could be much, much higher.

Why don't doctors give carbon dioxide, rather than oxygen? Why don't they issue carbon dioxide inhalers?

Quite simply, the reason is that doctors have not been trained to understand the importance and benefits of carbon dioxide. Ironically, about 40 years ago, some doctors did administer small amounts of carbon dioxide to asthmatics and emphysemics. But with the development of steroid drugs came the conviction that the new wonder drugs would always come to the rescue. Carbon dioxide use was discontinued.

Why should we sleep on the left side?

Although the lung capacity is slightly larger on one side than the other, there is no scientific evidence to explain why sleeping on the left side is better. Professor Buteyko simply observed over many years and work with tens of thousands of patients that those who slept on their left sides lost much less carbon dioxide than the others. The results are conclusive enough to make us urge you to arrange your pillow so that you sleep on your left side. You will certainly make up your own mind about this once you have experienced less hyperventilation during sleep.

Is the Breath Connection program helpful for those with degenerative conditions such as arthritis, rheumatism, and heart disease?

Certainly. Check the list of disorders that Breath Connection can help with, in Appendix B.

Should I do the Breath Connection program if I am pregnant?

Yes, the program is very helpful, and it can be especially useful if you suffer from antenatal sickness and postnatal depression. Reconditioning your breathing is beneficial to your developing baby, which is likely to be bigger and healthier as a result.

I have a young baby. What can I do for her?

Attend a Breath Connection workshop if you can, in order to learn how to help your baby. If you can't, read this book carefully and make notes for yourself if you think that would be helpful. Refer especially to the chapter on asthma and childhood. Obviously, placing tape over a baby's mouth as it sleeps is not always going to be a practical option. Do, however, try to close your baby's mouth with your finger when you see her breathing with an open mouth.

Asthma is very difficult to diagnose in young infants. If you know or suspect that you or your partner carry the gene that makes you more susceptible to asthma, be particularly watchful until your baby is old enough to be diagnosed. In the meantime, take practical measures such as reducing dairy foods, taking care to substitute other forms of calcium (see page 192).

Isn't carbon dioxide meant to be poisonous?

Our air contains about 200 times less carbon dioxide than we need to function effectively. That's why the alveoli of the lungs work so hard to make up this deficit by producing enough carbon dioxide for us. It is a myth that it is a damaging waste gas.

Which illnesses cannot be treated by Breath Connection?

At the end of Appendix B, you'll find a short list of conditions that don't, sadly, respond to the Breath Connection treatment because they are not caused by hyperventilation. Ninety percent of the illnesses to which we are prey can be alleviated by the Breath Connection techniques.

Do the Breathing Exercises prevent common colds and flu?

Yes, because they boost your immune system, which means that you will be less susceptible to infection. If you had flu or a cold before embarking on the Breath Connection program, we suggest that you take extra vitamin C, the herb Echinacea, and the mineral zinc. Your doctor or Breath Connection practitioner, who is aware of your personal profile, may offer more specific advice.

Some self-help/relaxation books recommend "retention breath," in which you breathe in, hold it, and then breathe out for a specified number of seconds. What do you think?

This may relax you, but it isn't helping your breathing or your health. If your Control Pause is 50 to 60 seconds, it doesn't matter how you breathe. With the Breath Connection method, the less time you take to breathe in the better, but it doesn't matter how long you take to breathe out.

Is it harmful for me to play the flute or sing?

If you are already hyperventilating and have a low Control Pause, we are sorry to say that it is harmful. As singing and playing wind instruments usually increase your rate of breathing, they are not recommended for anyone with a hyperventilation problem. You should, however, be fine if your Control Pause is high, and you have been balancing your breathing for a while. It is, really, only a question of setting aside your music for a short time. After getting the balance right, you can return to it and your carbon dioxide levels won't be affected enough to worry about. Of course, if you are a professional musician who needs to practice as well as perform under pressure, you may need to seek more specific advice.

What's wrong with the old-fashioned method of breathing into a brown paper bag, and then inhaling to reabsorb the carbon dioxide, especially if I am having a panic attack?

Nothing at all, and many asthmatics have also found it useful during attacks. Some hospitals also use the technique. Remember, however, that it is a quick fix—no more and no less. It will not deal with the root of your problem—hyperventilation.

Once I have learned the Breath Connection methods, will I be able to teach them to others?

No. Don't be misled by the apparent simplicity of our courses. Breath Connection practitioners all have a very sophisticated understanding of every complexity of breathing and its functions. All of our practitioners have been personally trained by Professor Buteyko and have up to 15 to 20 years of experience in teaching his methods.

Can I, as an asthmatic, go scuba diving or go in for other water sports that involve oxygen masks?

You need to check with a Breath Connection practitioner, or your doctor. It depends entirely on your Control Pause.

What are the dangers of developing osteoporosis if I cut down on dairy products, including milk?

See our section on diet and nutrition (page 187). Many other foods offer lots of calcium, including leafy green vegetables, cereals, some fruit, offal, pulses, and tofu.

When can I stop taking steroids?

Only when your Breath Connection practitioner and doctor recommend it.

Are the side effects of steroids reversible?

Yes. Following the Breath Connection program has a profound effect on all of your body systems and can lead to a reversal of all steroid side effects.

What about alcohol on the program?

Avoid it completely, if possible. Remember that the original course is only five days! If that's difficult, cut back to a maximum of two glasses of wine a day with meals. Remember that the Breath Connection program is essentially a holistic one, and you will obtain the greatest range of benefits if you undertake it with your whole health in mind. Aim for positive change all around.

Does that mean I should stop smoking?

You should not smoke while you are involved with the program and, in fact, Breath Connection offers an ideal kick start to a delayed resolve to quit. But we are not judgmental, and we realize that for many people the stress of giving up smoking leads them to overbreathe even more. Focusing on shallow breathing will certainly help you, but you may find hypnosis or acupuncture useful if you want to stop smoking.

Will Breath Connection help with my depression?

Absolutely, yes. It is not just your physical health that the program addresses. Your brain function, emotional and mental states, and instabilities are all addressed. Apart from anything else, you now know that you have taken control, and you have been empowered to do so. This action is almost always uplifting and self-affirming. However, remember that depression is a very complex illness and for some people specialist psychological or psychiatric help may be necessary.

Are the breathing exercises a form of stress management, then?

If you like, yes. Do the Control Pause for a few minutes and your shallow breathing will counteract any negative stress responses that your body produces. Use the Control Pause as a regular basic health and stress-level check.

Does Breath Connection work for genetic disorders?

Sometimes it can, as in the case of cystic fibrosis, for example. Refer to Appendix B.

Is it all right to sleep with plants and flowers in the room?

It's best if you don't. Plants and flowers eat carbon dioxide at night.

Is fasting a good idea?

In general, yes. Think of it as giving your body a holiday from the hard work of digestion, so that it can concentrate on eliminating toxins. Toxins are excreted through the pores of the skin, as well as through the bowel and in the urine. Over the centuries, many advanced societies have advocated occasional fasting. Some claim that the head is cleared and lightened (or enlightened!) as the body rests and clears itself. If you do fast, drink lots of water and organic carrot and beetroot juice. If you merely want to reduce your intake of solids, keep to a diet of light salads without oil, and fruit and vegetables. Raw vegetables are best. You can, if you wish, simply eat boiled rice.

As the body flushes away its waste, you may find that you get headaches, some mild diarrhea, and your breath may smell bad. These are all normal symptoms and act as evidence of the fact that your body is detoxifying. Drink plenty of water to flush the toxins, and try colonic irrigation, which also speeds up the process.

It is generally advised that you discuss any proposed fast with your doctor, particularly if you intend to fast for more than one or two days. If you have certain physical or emotional problems, it might be best to wait until you are stronger. No diabetic or hypoglycemic, for example, should ever fast. Other people should only do so when they have been advised that it is the right time, or optimal point, to embark on this useful cleansing exercise.

Can I be really tiresome and ask you to spell out for me, one more time, how I, as an asthmatic, should program my day?

Your question isn't tiresome at all. We encourage people to be at ease and confident about what they are undertaking with Breath Connection.

- Just after waking, hold your breath and sit up. Breathe gently through the nose and resist any desire to clear the chest by coughing. Try to retain your phlegm and release it in one go later. A violent coughing fit could lead to a full-blown asthma attack. Use the anticoughing techniques if necessary (see page 120).

- Whatever you used to do first in the morning, do it second. Your breathing comes first. An asthmatic's Control Pause is at its lowest, and the danger of hyperventilation is at its height, early in the morning.

- Do your breathing exercises and note down the figures. Allow 20 to 30 minutes for this.

- Take your medication (steroids) but avoid bronchodilators. It could be the mistake of your life—literally—to take relievers without immediate need. Many people—including athletes—do this, but it can worsen the situation in the long term.

- Do not use your peak flow meter. It is merely a register of symptoms.

- Don't eat breakfast unless you are hungry. You risk hyperventilation if you do so. Remember that food is also a reliever, and you should only take it if you need relief from hunger.

- Try to breathe shallowly on the way to work, whether you walk, ride, or drive.
- Do your Breath Connection exercises before lunch. Many people hyperventilate at mealtimes, not because of what or how much they eat, but how they do so.
- Check your Control Pause several times a day.
- Use your spare time—in the car, on a bus, in a restaurant, between meetings, while cooking—to shallow breathe. If you do hyperventilate, it will be easier to control. You could check that your breathing is appropriately light by holding the flame of a lighter beneath your nose. It should barely flicker.
- For those of you who ask which part of the lung you should use for breathing, the answer is the tip of your nose! Imagine that you don't have lungs at all. That way, ironically, they will function well.
- When going out into the cold from a warm room, or vice versa, breathe out just before opening the door, and then take five or 10 steps without breathing at all. Then breathe shallowly. This exercise will help you to avoid an asthma attack.
- If you enjoy sports and exercise, treat yourself! An active lifestyle—even for asthmatics—is far better than an overprotected one. But make sensible preparations. Exercising early in the morning is a good start to the day.
- Do your Breath Connection exercises before dinner.
- Before you sleep, do a Control Pause. Tape up your mouth, settle yourself on your left side, and enjoy the best sleep you've had in years.

16

Science and History

Now that you know Breath Connection works, you might like to learn a little more about why it works and how it was developed.

You know that over 200 illnesses and disorders can be successfully treated by Breath Connection. You know that results are fast, techniques are simple and inexpensive, and seldom drug-dependent. You know that the reconditioning of your breathing and a proper understanding of the vital importance of carbon dioxide is crucial to your health. But how did Professor Buteyko know this when he first began to develop his research in Russia just after the Second World War?

Early in 1960, having endured years when his work was underfunded, if not dismissed outright, Professor Buteyko announced his findings to a forum at the Institute of Experimental Biology and Medicine at the Siberian branch of the then USSR's Academy of Science. Despite encountering initial skepticism, he was allowed to continue with his work and is fully recognized today by his government.

Studies across Russia and in Australia have shown anyone following the Buteyko techniques will benefit and that 90 percent of asthmatics reduce their drug dependency. Both frequency and severity of asthmatic attacks are diminished by natural means. His methods have proved to be a near-infallible way of monitoring general health and of improving quality of all-around health. To date, over a million asthmatics in Russia have benefited from his techniques. And most of them are no longer dependent upon medication of any kind.

Despite vast amounts of money thrown at research into respiratory and other illnesses, few conventional Western approaches have come close to dealing so effectively with asthma, cancers, arthritis, and other degenerative diseases. Symptomatic relief, which requires continued use of new drugs, has been developed but the fundamental problems of asthma and other respiratory disorders have not been addressed. We may be living longer and even have the material comforts that should allow us to enjoy comfortable old age, but for many people their final years—even their middle age—are severely limited by a degenerative disease.

As yet, most of us only seek medical advice when we know we are ill. Then we may be prescribed drugs that we may be expected to take for the rest of our lives. The Breath Connection methods turn this whole idea on its head. Why wait until something goes wrong or breaks down before looking after your body? It's simple. All you need to do is learn to breathe properly.

So why has it taken so long for Professor Buteyko's principles to be embraced here in the West? We tentatively offer an analogy with Copernicus (1473–1543). Before his time, even the most brilliant of Renaissance thinkers believed that the sun and the other planets revolved around the earth. A century later, Galileo, who advanced Copernicus's pioneering theories, was similarly pilloried. In the West today, our understanding of respiratory medicine is still very limited: Few orthodox practitioners realize that so many disorders are connected to incorrect breathing, not simply the obvious illnesses of the breathing tracts and lungs.

At Breath Connection, we operate from scientific foundations. Konstantin Buteyko is a professor of conventional medicine and trained within rigorous scientific disciplines. While recognizing the importance of complementary and alternative medicine, we don't reject established understandings of the way the human body works. It is our hope and belief that the Buteyko principles themselves will soon be regarded as conventional. Bear in mind that Professor Buteyko's work was conducted at a time when the dissemination of ideas from East to West was slower than it is today. It first came to attention outside Russia when one of the professor's chief associates began to demonstrate the importance of Professor Buteyko's ideas and methods in the Western world.

Hyperventilation, or overbreathing as it was known in the nineteenth century, is the simple cause of a huge raft of illnesses. We hope that our book has overturned that raft and shown that shallow breathing, rather than taking deep breaths, is a first principle for permanent good health—whatever your age when you begin to practice it. Hyperventilation is the cause of illness, not a result of it. Be spare with your air. Deep breaths can lead to deep trouble. We respect the other elements—fire, water, and earth—rather more than we have hitherto respected the fourth, air. Just as fire can comfort and help to nourish us but also damage us if it is not controlled, and just as we know that a deprivation of sunlight can cause SAD (Seasonal Affective Disorder) in some people, we should be aware that our consumption of air should also be controlled. Too much air breathed in can be as damaging as, or more damaging than, too much ultraviolet light. We know that we can survive, if we must, without food or water for long periods. Yogis have used deprivation to heighten spiritual experiences. But we are mistaken if we ignore or neglect to monitor the amount of the air we take in and underestimate the value of carbon dioxide.

The regime we offer is not merely about common sense and personal responsibility, however. It is about choice. There is usually a hard way and an easy way to confront every one of life's dilemmas. We hope that we will have shown you that the 'helpful' discipline of Breath Connection pays an immediate dividend. Your life will become easier. You can stop fearing allergies, panic attacks, and insomnia, chronic fatigue, and arthritis as well as conditions most often associated with a disorder of the breathing apparatus.

And all this is due to work and research doggedly pursued by Professor Buteyko years before he had any real hope of his findings being accepted.

Breath control was actually understood over 3,000 years ago in Tibet, where they believed that death entered a person through the mouth. Much later the Romans employed the same word for *breath* and *spirit*. In Sanskrit, *prana* means not only breath but universal life force. Recently, here in the West, it has been observed that creatures, such as mice, who breathe rapidly have shorter life spans than those, such as elephants, who breathe slowly. Such findings have contributed to a universal and timeless debate about how the very act of breathing influences how we expend an allotted life force. These same findings have also served to confuse as they tend to correlate slow breathing with deep breathing and a long, healthy life.

Regulating our breathing conditions all the body's systems, as we have shown, and is a basic form of meditation which can reduce stress as well as beneficially affect physical disorder. But meditation as such should not be confused with the Breath Connection program. Although it can be generally helpful, it does not offer specific help in dealing with disease, as Breath Connection does. We embrace the mind-body holistic principles alongside practical and designated aims and techniques for patients who are or may become ill. We are not in the business of restoring inner calm, in the same way that a meditational program might be.

A hundred years ago, two Austrian scientists, Breyer and Gering, discovered that humans were the only species on earth who had not developed a correct way to breathe. Not much happened after this pioneering finding. Fast-forward several decades to the earliest findings of Professor Buteyko, who began to see that most humans were taking in up to 4 to 10 times more air than they needed and, moreover, saw the link between overbreathing and a huge list of diseases that many before him had seen as being not only chronic and debilitating, but incurable. With generous and proper respect, he acknowledged the pioneering work of Verigo and Bohr (see page 240).

This had helped him to see that when too much air was drawn deep into the lungs, carbon dioxide was then being exhaled in great quantity rather than being retained to facilitate the oxygen's work. Professor Buteyko began to encounter the old chestnut about oxygen being good for us—and so the more the better, please—and carbon dioxide being a poisonous waste gas.

When the human biological system was developing, aeons ago, the air contained a percentage of CO_2 at least a hundred times higher than it is today. But this level has been steadily depleted by the natural development of the environment, including the culture of trees and plants which absorb carbon dioxide. The percentage of CO_2 in today's air is less than one-half of 1 percent. In the months we spend awaiting birth in the womb, we get used to absorbing a gaseous mix which contains seven to eight percent carbon dioxide. What a shock to be born into such a differently balanced gaseous environment and how unnecessary it has been to routinely smack the newborn's bottom, causing him or her to gulp in a lungful of alien air.

The alveoli in the lungs have adapted resourcefully to this situation, as we have seen, and create an environment of 6.5 percent carbon dioxide within the body, but we still need to breathe correctly to maintain this level, and asthmatics and those people with some other illnesses find this difficult. When the carbon dioxide level in the body sinks below 3.5 percent, palpitations, dizziness, and wheezing occur. Breath Connection simply teaches you to normalize the carbon dioxide levels up to about 6 percent, which is our human physiological norm.

Science, as we understand the word, didn't exist as a discipline for study until the early eighteenth century. Until then, ideas about the world's mysteries were largely influenced by religious and spiritual beliefs. Many of these still prevail. Breathing used to be considered a means of cooling the blood. The ideas of the French chemist, Antoine Lavoisier (1743–1794), who saw oxygen as a great life force and carbon dioxide as a poison, are still widely accepted. His experiments with mice placed under glass domes along with a burning candle supported his view when the candle and mouse expired at roughly the same time as the oxygen supply was exhausted. Because only carbon dioxide remained, he concluded that it must be a poison.

In 1909, Professor Yandell Henderson at Yale University dared to disagree and said that "oxygen is in no sense a stimulant to living creatures" after he had observed that it was in fact a carbon dioxide deficiency that caused animals forced to breathe in experimental conditions to die. Few listened to him.

The toxicity of oxygen had been observed as early as 1899, but it was not until the 1960s that scientists, such as the young Professor Buteyko, began to understand it. Some premature babies who breathed in 100 percent oxygen during incubation developed a form of blindness known as retrolensil fibroplasia.

Even the most brilliant of scientists cannot change the composition of our atmosphere, which currently contains twice as much oxygen as we need to function well and 200 times less carbon dioxide. But many are now continuing Professor Buteyko's precepts and working with the adaptability and ingenuity of the human body to ensure that we control the elements of our air so that it suits us and our environment.

Overbreathing, or hyperventilation, was first identified in 1871 by the American physician da Costa, who observed the palpitations, coughing, and breathlessness, coupled with stress, from which many soldiers returning from the American Civil War suffered. His observations were studied later by the British doctor John Haldane, whose work on a large group of healthy soldiers set out the norms for breathing. We should breathe four to six liters of air into the lungs every minute. The norms are still in use today. Haldane recognized the importance of the balance between oxygen and carbon dioxide in the breathing process.

In 1905, the Russian physiologist, Verigo, and the Dutch physicist, Bohr, independently built on Haldane's work, demonstrating yet again the wonderful international chair of scientific and medical progress. They ascertained that without carbon dioxide in the body, oxygen cannot perform its regenerative function and, moreover, blood pressure will increase. Yet many hospitals still automatically pump asthma patients, admitted in crisis, with oxygen which they don't require and which can exacerbate their condition.

It was against this dawning of understanding that Professor Buteyko trained as a doctor in Russia and formed his interest in respiratory and related disorders. He came to realize that none of us needs to breathe in large amounts of air or compete with the stopwatch and breathe a set number of times each minute. He saw the dangers of hyperventilation, and he realized that taking in more than four to six liters of air per minute wrongly filled the lungs with an unnecessary amount of air. The central nervous system can be destabilized, and the digestive, hormonal, elimination, immune, and cardiovascular systems damaged. Fatigue and general weakness also occur. For Professor Buteyko, it became a matter of training patients to breathe deeply in order to witness the results. He then had to prove to other doctors that patients who were inhaling as much as 10 to 15 liters of air each minute were damaging their health.

He had noticed that patients' breathing often became deeper as the onset of death approached and he learned to judge very accurately how long someone had to live simply by monitoring his or her breathing. His passion for the study of respiratory disorder was awakened when he was a third-year medical student. He noticed that patients who were hyperventilating recovered if their breathing was encouraged to be more shallow. The first seedlings of today's knowledge about how correct breathing can affect many nonrespiratory illnesses were planted at this time, along with the early formation of Professor Buteyko's philosophy about diet and stress management. At first subjected to ridicule, Buteyko's ideas were eventually accepted by the Russian Ministry of Health, but it was to be years before his efforts were properly funded, recognized, and adopted throughout the Soviet Union.

Men—and women—of science who are ahead of their time, such as Joseph Lister, whose findings created the foundation for modern anesthetics, and Louis Pasteur, who taught the world about the importance of antiseptics, suffered the indignity of having much of their work ridiculed or unrecognized throughout their lifetimes. At least Professor Buteyko has lived to see his ideas widely accepted and adopted in Russia. A 95 percent success rate for his methods is recorded in Russia, and the remaining 5 percent of patients enjoy at least some relief if not a complete cure.

This book is about the importance of breath in our lives. It is so much more than a set of breathing exercises and a technique for hyperventilation. Nearly half a century of medical research and experience by Professor Buteyko has created a new medical system which addresses the relationship between oxygen and carbon dioxide in our bodies, thereby providing the key to our physical and mental health.

We at Breath Connection are very proud to be involved in the advancement of Professor Buteyko's life-saving message and hope that it will be a very short time before its obvious simplicity and effectiveness are regarded as the norm. Just as the achievements of Lister, Pasteur, and other scientific geniuses have formed the cornerstones of our modern concept of good health, Professor Buteyko and his revolutionary approach will form one of the vital foundations of our health in the future.

Appendix A: Recordkeeping Charts

BREATH CONNECTION WEEKLY PROGRAM FOR MILD ASTHMA: RECORDKEEPING CHART

Date	Time	Start Pulse	Control Pause	Shallow Breathe	Control Pause	Shallow Breathe	Control Pause + 5 seconds	Shallow Breathe	Control Pause + 10 seconds	Shallow Breathe	Control Pause	Final Pulse	Medication Intake and Physical Condition
	Morning												
	Afternoon												
	Evening												
	Morning												
	Afternoon												
	Evening												
	Morning												
	Afternoon												
	Evening												
	Morning												
	Afternoon												
	Evening												
	Morning												
	Afternoon												
	Evening												
	Morning												
	Afternoon												
	Evening												
	Morning												
	Afternoon												
	Evening												

BREATH CONNECTION WEEKLY PROGRAM FOR SEVERE ASTHMA: RECORDKEEPING CHART

Date	Time	Check Pulse	Control Pause	Decrease Breathing	Control Pause	Rest	Control Pause	Decrease Breathing	Control Pause	Rest	Control Pause
	Mor										
	Aft										
	Eve										
	Mor										
	Aft										
	Eve										
	Mor										
	Aft										
	Eve										
	Mor										
	Aft										
	Eve										
	Mor										
	Aft										
	Eve										
	Mor										
	Aft										
	Eve										

Do this exercise 3 times a day. For further instructions regarding continuation of practice, see chapter

Decrease Breathing	Control Pause	Rest	Control Pause	Decrease Breathing	Control Pause	Rest	Control Pause	Decrease Breathing	Control Pause	Rest	Final Pulse	Medication Intake and Physical Condition

BREATH CONNECTION WEEKLY PROGRAM FOR MILD–SEVERE EMPHYSEMA: RECORDKEEPING CHART

Date	Time	Start Pulse	Control Pause	Shallow Breathe	Control Pause + 5 seconds	Final Pulse	Intake of Medication and Physical Condition
	Morning						
	Afternoon						
	Evening						
	Morning						
	Afternoon						
	Evening						
	Morning						
	Afternoon						
	Evening						
	Morning						
	Afternoon						
	Evening						
	Morning						
	Afternoon						
	Evening						
	Morning						
	Afternoon						
	Evening						
	Morning						
	Afternoon						
	Evening						

BREATH CONNECTION WEEKLY EXERCISE PROGRAM FOR SEVERE EMPHYSEMA: RECORDKEEPING CHART

Date	Time	Start Pulse	Control Pause	Exercises 1, 2, and 3	Control Pause	Final Pulse	Intake of Medication and Physical Condition
	Morning						
	Afternoon						
	Evening						
	Before Sleep						
	Morning						
	Afternoon						
	Evening						
	Before Sleep						
	Morning						
	Afternoon						
	Evening						
	Before Sleep						
	Morning						
	Afternoon						
	Evening						
	Before Sleep						
	Morning						
	Afternoon						
	Evening						
	Before Sleep						
	Morning						

BREATH CONNECTION WEEKLY PROGRAM FOR COLDS, FLU, AND HAYFEVER: RECORDKEEPING CHART

Date	Time	First Pulse	Control Pause	Shallow Breathe	Control Pause	Shallow Breathe	Control Pause	Shallow Breathe	Control Pause	Final Pulse	Intake of Medication and Physical Condition
	Morning										
	Afternoon										
	Evening										
	Morning										
	Afternoon										
	Evening										
	Morning										
	Afternoon										
	Evening										
	Morning										
	Afternoon										
	Evening										
	Morning										
	Afternoon										
	Evening										

BREATH CONNECTION WEEKLY SELF-CARE PROGRAM FOR STRESS AND BRONCHITIS: RECORDKEEPING CHART

Date	Time	Start Pulse	Control Pause	Shallow Breathe	Control Pause	Final Pulse	Intake of Medication and Physical Condition
	Morning						
	1 hour before sleep						
	Morning						
	1 hour before sleep						
	Morning						
	1 hour before sleep						
	Morning						
	1 hour before sleep						
	Morning						
	1 hour before sleep						
	Morning						
	1 hour before sleep						

249

BREATH CONNECTION WEEKLY BRONCHITIS PROGRAM: RECORDKEEPING CHART

Date	Time	Start Pulse	Control Pause	Shallow Breathe	Control Pause	Final Pulse	Intake of Medication and Physical Condition
	Morning						
	1 hour before sleep						
	Morning						
	1 hour before sleep						
	Morning						
	1 hour before sleep						
	Morning						
	1 hour before sleep						
	Morning						
	1 hour before sleep						
	Morning						
	1 hour before sleep						

BREATH CONNECTION WEEKLY PROGRAM FOR CHILDREN WITH ASTHMA AND BRONCHITIS: RECORDKEEPING CHART

Date	Time	Start Pulse	Control Pause	Number of Steps	Minutes of Shallow Breathing	Intake of Medication and Physical Condition
	Morning					
	Afternoon					
	Evening					
	Morning					
	Afternoon					
	Evening					
	Morning					
	Afternoon					
	Evening					
	Morning					
	Afternoon					
	Evening					
	Morning					
	Afternoon					
	Evening					
	Morning					
	Afternoon					
	Evening					
	Morning					
	Afternoon					
	Evening					

BREATH CONNECTION PROGRAM FOR SPORTS: RECORDKEEPING CHART

Date	Time	First Pulse	Control Pause	Shallow Breathe	Pulse	Control Pause	Shallow Breathe	Control Pause	Pulse	Intake of Medication and Physical Condition
	Before Sport									
	After Sport									
	Before Sport									
	After Sport									
	Before Sport									
	After Sport									
	Before Sport									
	After Sport									
	Before Sport									
	After Sport									
	Before Sport									
	After Sport									
	Before Sport									
	After Sport									

Appendix B: Most Common Health Problems and Symptoms That Can Be Treated by Breath Connection

Acidosis aklalosis

Agoraphobia

AIDS*

Allergies*

Anemia*

Anorexia nervosa*

Apathy

Arthritis (osteo and rheuma-
toid)*

Asthma attacks

Bed-wetting

Breathing without pause after
exhaling

Breathlessness

Bronchitis

Bulimia*

Cancer*

Cerebral palsy*

Chest pains (not in the heart
region)*

Chronic blocked nose

Chronic diarrhea

Chronic fatigue syndrome*

Chronic pneumonia*

Circulation problems*

Colds

Concentration problems

Constipation

Coughing

Cystic Fibrosis*

Depression*

Deterioration of vision

Diarrhea

Dizziness

Drug addiction*

Dry skin

Eczema

Edema

Epilepsy*

Far-sightedness

Fear without reason

Flatulence

Flu

Frigidity

Gulf War Syndrome*

Gynecological problems*

Hay Fever

Headaches

Heart attacks*

Heart conditions*

Heartburn

High blood pressure*

Hyperventilation

Impotence (male)

Infertility*

Insomnia*

Insulin-dependent diabetes*

Irritable bowel syndrome

Irritability

Itching

Kidney disease*

Lack of concentration

Loss of feeling in the limbs*

Loss of memory

Low blood pressure*

Memory loss

Menopause symptoms*

Mental fatigue

Migraine*

Multiple sclerosis (MS)*

Muscle pains

Nightmares

Pain in the heart region*

Painful and irregular periods* (female)

Palpitations*

Panic attacks

Parkinson's disease*

Post- and prenatal depression*

Posttrauma stress*

Premenstrual syndrom (PMS)*

Rhinitis

Scleroderma*

Short temper

Shortness of breath

Sinusitis

Skin problems*

Sleep apnea*

Snoring

Spasms of brain/heart/kidney/ extremities/blood vessels*

Sterility*

Stomach sickness

Stress

Stroke*

Thyroid problems*

Tightness around chest

Trembling and tics*

Ulcers*

Varicose veins

Weight gain

Weight loss

The preceding list represents 90 of the 200 illnesses that Professor Buteyko discovered to be caused by hyperventilation. More than 90 percent of us suffer from these illnesses. When Professor Buteyko trained his patients to stop hyperventilating, their conditions either improved considerably or disappeared completely.

Anyone who suffers from asthma, emphysema, or bronchitis and one of the asterisked conditions (see above), is advised not to undertake the self-care programs in this book. You can still benefit from the Breath Connection program, but we strongly recommend that you do so under the guidance of a fully qualified and experienced Breath Connection practitioner. These illnesses are more difficult to treat and require a very individual approach for each patient. Although they will not be cured within a week, you should experience some improvement in your symptoms within a short period of time. You will, however, have to practice for some time, to remove the root cause of the condition.

Illnesses That Cannot Be Helped by Breath Connection

There are some illnesses that cannot be treated by Breath Connection. The most commonly known of these include the following:

Alzheimer's disease (although it can help in the early stages)
Autism
Back pain
Bad posture
Coma
Manic depression
Psoriasis
Psychosis
Schizophrenia
Tonsillitis
Trauma/Accidents

Appendix C: Glossary

Acid/Alkaline balance: Otherwise known as the pH balance. This is the ratio of acids to alkalis measured in body fluids such as blood, gastric juices, and urine. Maintaining the correct pH value is essential for the normal, healthy functioning of every cell in the body. This balance, or homeostasis, can be detrimentally affected by a poor diet (including too much protein, sugar, or grains), stress, and hyperventilation.

Asthma: An inflammatory disease of the airways, resulting in bronchospasm attacks that induce coughing, wheezing, and gasping for air, among other symptoms.

Allergy: A defensive response by the body to a normally harmless trigger or allergen. Common allergens include foods, pollens, metals, household chemicals, dust mites, feathers, and animal fur. An allergy is an abnormal response, which indicates that the body is in a hypersensitive state.

Alveoli: Clusters of air sacs that are responsible for the exchange of gases between the lungs and the bloodstream.

Balanced breathing: Slow, shallow breathing that balances the delicate ratio of carbon dioxide to oxygen in the lungs and ensures optimum health.

Bronchitis: The inflammation of the mucous membranes of the respiratory system.

Bronchodilator: A drug taken by patients with respiratory conditions such as asthma. Bronchodilators artificially dilate the bronchial tubes in order to facilitate breathing. However, by forcing a greater intake of oxygen into the lungs, these drugs further exacerbate hyperventilation, leading to a greater deterioration of the patient's medical condition.

Carbon dioxide: A natural gas, and the body's own, natural bronchodilator. In its various chemical forms, carbon dioxide (also known as CO_2) is responsible for maintaining the correct pH balance of the blood and is a vital regulator of the body's systems.

Control Pause: A technique that allows you to measure the level of carbon dioxide in your lungs, and hence the state of your present (and future) health.

Emphysema: A severe respiratory condition in which the alveoli (air sacs) of the lungs fail to contract properly, thereby failing to expel sufficient air. This results in constant breathing difficulties, including serious shortness of breath.

Hyperventilation: Hyperventilation, or overbreathing, occurs when the intake of air is greater than the physiological norm of 5 liters per minute. This lowers the level of carbon dioxide in the bloodstream, which subsequently deprives the tissues of essential oxygen. According to Professor Buteyko, hyperventilation is a breathing disorder that causes a wide range of illnesses and is not merely a symptom of these illnesses.

Immune system: The body's overall defense system against internal and external attack. The immune system produces antibodies that help to protect the body against foreign substances and encourages the healing mechanism. A strong immune system deals with invaders, such as bacteria or viruses, quickly and efficiently.

Nebulizer: A method of administering bronchodilator drugs in very high doses.

Overbreathing: *See* Hyperventilation.

Oxygenation: The vital transportation of oxygen through the bloodstream, from the lungs to the body tissues.

Peak flow meter: An instrument used by the conventional medical profession to measure lung capacity.

pH: *See* Acid/Alkaline balance.

Respiration: The overall exchange of oxygen and carbon dioxide between the atmosphere, blood, lungs, and body cells.

Spasm: An uncontrollable contraction of one or more muscles. A spasm is one example of the body's natural defense mechanism against excessive loss of carbon dioxide.

Steroid: Natural steroids are chemicals such as cholesterol and hormones that are released by certain glands in the body. Steroids are also artificially manufactured, in order to mimic the actions of the body's own natural steroids. Artificial steroids are used preventatively for the treatment of asthma and other respiratory disorders, among other things.

Appendix D: Resources

Breath Connection U.S.	350 East 54 Street, New York, NY 10022-5049
Telephone:	Information on courses: Toll free: 1-800-259-4644
Fax:	212-415-9060
E-mail:	admin@breathconnection.com
Web site:	http://www.breathconnection.com
Telephone Advisory Service:	Contact email admin@breathconnection.com for further information
The Hale Clinic	7 Park Crescent, London W1N 3HE
Telephone	011 44 171 631 0156
Fax:	011 44 171 323 1693
Web site:	http://www.haleclinic.com
E-mail:	admin@haleclinic.com

Bibliography

Burne, Jerome. "Hyperventilation: The New Argument about Asthma," *Independent on Sunday,* 5 October 1997.

Carola, Robert, et al. *Human Anatomy and Physiology,* 2nd edition. New York: McGraw-Hill, 1992.

Chopra, Deepak. *Boundless Energy.* Rider, 1995.

Graham, Tess. "Self-Management of Asthma through Normalisation of Breathing: The Role of Breathing Therapy," *Australian Medical Journal,* December 1998.

Hale, Teresa. *The Hale Clinic Guide to Good Health.* Kyle Cathie Books, 1996.

Holford, Patrick. *The Optimum Nutrition Bible.* Piatkus, 1997.

Kenton, Leslie. *The New Ageless Ageing.* Vermilion, 1995.

McCance, Kathryn L., and Sue E. Heuther. *Pathophysiology: The Biologic Basis for Disease in Adults and Children,* 2nd edition. Mosby-Year Book Inc., 1994.

May-Ropers, Christine, and David Schweitzer. *Never Acidic Again.*

Perera, Judith. "The Hazards of Heavy Breathing," *New Scientist,* 3 December 1988.

Price, Sylvia, and Lorraine Wilson. *Clinical Concepts of Disease Processes,* 4th edition. Mosby-Year Book Inc., 1972.

Rowett, H. G. Q., *Basic Anatomy and Physiology,* 3rd edition. John Murray (Publishers) Ltd., 1988.

Shivapremananda, Swami. *Yoga for Stress Relief.* Gaia Books, 1997.

The Sivananda Yoga Centre. *The Book of Yoga: The Complete Step-by-Step Guide,* Ebury Press, 1983.

Stalmatski, Alexander. *Freedom from Asthma.* Kyle Cathie Books, 1997.

Weil, Andrew. *Spontaneous Healing.* Little Brown & Co., 1995.

Index

abdominal breathing exercises, for panic attacks, 123
accidents, 255
aches and pains, 126, 132, 254
    see also pain
acid/alkaline balance, see pH balance
acidosis alkalosis, 177, 253
acquired immune deficiency syndrome, see AIDS
acupuncture, 21, 26, 27
    for smoking cessation, 230
adrenal cortex, and steroid use, 68
adrenaline, treatment with, 61, 62, 66
    and asthma-related deaths, 65
aging, premature, 179
agoraphobia, 186, 253
agrochemicals, 30, 128, 179
AIDS, 19, 184, 185, 253
air intake, ideal, 33, 47, 240
    see also inhalation
air travel, 74, 89, 201
alcohol use
    and elimination system, 128
    to handle stress, 125
    reducing, 164, 166, 193, 203, 229–30

allergens
    and asthma, 168
    inhaling, 171
allergies, 180, 182, 184, 253
    Breath Connection effect on, 22, 83
    as defense mechanism, 143
    to food, 30, 184
    and pH balance, 166
    suppression of, 62
    susceptibility to, 40, 171, 178, 184
alternative medicine, 6, 12, 236
    see also complementary medicine
alveoli, 36, 227, 239
    in emphysema, 103
    during hyperventilation, 167
Alzheimer's disease, 255
amino acids, 190
aminophylline, 65
anabolic steroids, 67
Andrews, Professor Gavin, 176
anemia, 253
anger, 186, 254
angina, 40, 162, 165, 175
animal hair, and asthma, 168
anorexia nervosa, 135, 166, 187, 253

from overbreathing, 171
reduction of, 62
steroids to treat, 67
influenza, *see* flu
inhalation
excessive, 45, 167, 171, 236,
240
optimum rate of, 47–9
process of, 36
rate of, for asthmatics, 33, 34
reduced air volume in, 80, 139,
219
to treat panic attack, 123
in yogic breathing, 221
inhaler, use of, 36, 64
by children, 151, 157
by mild asthmatics, 78
by severe asthmatics, 86, 91
insomnia, 39, 167, 172, 180, 185,
254
Institute for Cosmic Medicine,
180
Institute of Experimental Biology
and Medicine, 234
insufflation cartridges, 64
Ipratropium bromide, 64
irritability, 39, 126, 180, 186, 254
irritable bowel syndrome, 177,
254
Isoprenaline, 64, 65
itching, 254

junk food
avoiding, 137, 147, 190, 215
in elimination system, 179

Karpov, Anatoly, 185
Ketotifen, 65
kidney
disease of, 87, 254
function of, 31, 37, 128, 179

Lavoisier, Antoine, 239
life expectancy, 28–31
and altitude, 104
and breathing rate, 237
for cancer patients, 204
for emphysemics, 101
increasing, 178
lifestyle
and asthma control, 89, 140, 233
changes to, 163, 195
as health consideration, 9, 35,
164
Lister, Joseph, 242
liver, function of, 30, 128, 179
Lowman, Al, 14
Lum, L., 181
lung(s), 36
breathing from, 219, 233
collapse of, 86
decreased use of, 91
in emphysema, 103
fibrosis in, 35–6, 118
inflammation of, 178
sclerosis in, 118
size of, 224–5
transplant of, 104, 105
lung capacity, 224, 225
in children, 159
in emphysema, 103, 105
reduced, from hyperventilation,
35

Ma Huang, 66
maintenance plan, 212–18
mealtimes, 189
guidelines for, 192–3
hyperventilation during, 233
meat, in diet, 164, 191, 192
medical insurance premiums, 22
medication, *see* drugs, pharmaceutical; *specific medications*

275

dysfunctional conditions of,
180–2
during panic attack, 123
neurons, 182
nightmares, 254
Norton, Dr. Richard, 170
Nutrition, 132
see also diet

obesity, Breath Connection effect
on, 13, 23, 166, 174, 183, 187
optimal health, 27
Osler, Sir William, 169
osteoporosis, 63, 92, 192, 229
ovaries, 182
overbreathing, *see* hyperventilation
overwork, 132
Oxitropium, 64
oxygen
in atmosphere, 162, 240
balance with carbon dioxide,
3–4, 28, 33–4, 45, 50, 77,
141, 178, 215, 240
brain need for, 176, 177
at high altitudes, 104, 180
inadequate, 37
from inhalation, 36–7
and muscles, 171, 172
and protein meals, 99, 190
requirement for, 2, 38, 47
for severely asthmatic children,
157
toxicity of, 239–40
use of, by emphysemics, 103–4
oxygen mask, sports involving, 229
oxyhemoglobin, 37

pain
chronic, 67
as illness signal, 132
relief from, 178
see also aches and pains

palpitations, 174, 175, 254
and carbon dioxide level, 181,
239
in panic attack, 122
pancreas
and carbon dioxide, 23
function of, 183
pH in, 177
panic attacks, 7, 122–5, 171, 182,
185
and carbon dioxide, 39
deep breath to relieve, 42, 123,
228
treatment for, 124–5, 254
panting, 35
paper bag, breathing into, 123,
228
paralysis, during sleep, 39
Parkinson's disease, 254
Pasteur, Louis, 242
peak flow meter, 72–3, 232
for asthmatic children, 147
peptic ulcers, 63
performance
of athletes, 23
Breath Connection effect on, 21
pesticides, 30, 179
pharmaceutical companies, 11, 77
pH balance
and allergies, 166
of blood, 177, 178
of human body, 37, 40, 178
phlegm
with bronchitis, 115
reducing, during sleep, 53
release of, 232
physiotherapy, 36
pineal gland, 31
pins and needles, as symptom, 172
Pirbuterol, 64
pituitary gland, 31, 182
placebo effect, 61